Expert Becoming a Dialysis Technician

Must Have Beginners Guide for Anyone Entering the Hemodialysis Technician Profession

Cassia Ann

ISBN 9798701241181

Chapter Beginning Quotes: Cassia Ann

Editor: Sharon Garner

Cover Design: *Digital_quasim*

Photographs: Cassia Ann & John Daryl, Illustrator

Definitions: Reprinted with permission from National Kidney Foundation, Inc.

DISCLAIMER

Cassia Ann is not claiming to represent any dialysis facility, company, or corporation. Cassia Ann has based her book on her opinions and experiences in working at many dialysis units all over New York City.

Every effort has been made to ensure that the information in this book is accurate and current at the time of publication. The author is not responsible for any misuse or misunderstanding of any information contained herein, or any loss, damage, or injury, be it health, financial, or otherwise, suffered by any individual or group acting upon or relying on information contained herein. None of the opinions or suggestions in this book is intended to replace medical protocol, medical opinions, or clinical mandates in the United States of America. If you have any concerns while working as a Dialysis Patient Care Technician, you should definitely request your unit's and state's protocols. None of this information is for definite intended use, being mere suggestions and opinions from author Cassia Ann. Names are sometimes changed to protect the identity of advisors.

DEDICATION

I dedicate this book to all new dialysis technicians, individuals interested in getting into dialysis work, and experienced technicians who desire to improve their patient care skills and techniques.

TABLE OF CONTENTS

PREFACE

I was inspired to write this book because I noticed as each year passed that it became harder and harder, for many reasons, for people to enter the dialysis technician field. I found that newbies and interested candidates didn't have available, a point of view from a hemodialysis technician currently in the field, who could explain what dialysis really is, what it takes to be a hemodialysis technician, the education requirements, the demands, the benefits, the pros and cons of the job, and so much more. I believe that if I had a guide like this when coming into the dialysis field, I definitely would've been farther ahead in my awareness of how to be absolutely professional and full of wisdom.

This book was written for those who have an interest in becoming a dialysis technician but are unsure how to go about preparing for and finding a job in the field. Or maybe you're someone who wants an overview on how to get your foot in the door, and how to appropriately handle patients with end stage renal failure.

By reading this book, you will equip yourself to understand the different fundamentals of working in a dialysis unit: the ups and downs (from my prospective); how to make your day productive; and what it's really like to work ten to thirteen hours a day, three days a week. Most of all, you'll explore my advice in deciding if this is the best career choice for you.

CHAPTER #1
HOW TO GET INTO THE
DIALYSIS PATIENT CARE
TECHNICIAN FIELD

There's no greater joy than discovering the benefits of something you love.

I want to congratulate you on your interest in the hemodialysis patient care technician field. By picking up this book, not only are you diving into my experience as a professional, but you are on your way to understanding what it takes to be a dedicated dialysis technician. This is an interesting but serious medical field. I am reminded of that each time I prepare to come to work. As I reflect on all my years as a technician, I realize many people have asked me how I became a dialysis technician and how they can become one.

This is definitely not a fly-by-night job, like a fast-food restaurant. It has become tougher to enter the dialysis field, and the standards have gotten higher. Please note that the dialysis field is very different now from the time I entered it. However, the benefits vary but are great overall for this occupation.

If you're coming out of dialysis school already state certified then you really don't have to worry about trying to get another certification other than CPR (cardiopulmonary resuscitation).

3

If you're coming into this field without any experience, or from a school that doesn't state certify you, it will require a huge amount of positive effort on your part to show the clinical manager that you are able to do the job, and that you are trainable. Depending on your facility, you may be given a choice of which state certification you would like to take. Later in this chapter I will discuss the two basic choices.

State certifications are no joke. People I knew and worked with lost their jobs around the time every dialysis technician in New York City had to be certified. They either couldn't pass the standards of the test, or refused to participate in the test for various reasons. If you're new to learning about dialysis, I emphasize over and over: Do your research on the aspects of end stage renal failure and dialysis. Search online for qualified dialysis websites, study and watch videos on how to prime a dialyzer, how to set up hemodialysis machines, and more.

Understand also that this book covers my experiences and gives my suggestions only. The dialysis world is constantly changing its protocols, standards, procedures, and the way they handle patients. That's why I stress in every chapter of this book that you check with your unit regarding every detail so you can provide the best services possible. Some clinics are extremely strict in their patient care procedures, and if you aren't careful you can be fired as quickly as you were hired—and possibly be banned from the dialysis field, depending on where you were hired. Some facilities maintain employee databases and are required to look up your file if another unit calls to check your qualifications for a patient care tech job. 4

If someone puts "don't rehire" in your file then that might cause issues with your new clinical job—they may not accept you with open arms. Be sure that if you decide to leave the nephrology field that you are in good standing. Several things are standard for becoming a dialysis technician: You must have deep, not surface (fake) empathy, understanding, a caring attitude, and patience. These people who receive in-center dialysis are human beings just like you and me. They may have families and other people relying on them, and they require care, concern, and professionalism.

Ask yourself these questions:

Can I handle seeing and dealing with a lot of blood?

Do I really have a passion to help sickly individuals?

Can I handle the death of a patient I may have constantly talked with?

Do I really have a desire to do this?

If you say "no" to any of those questions, this isn't for you.

Dialysis as a Job or a Career

Decide in the beginning stages of pursuing work in dialysis whether you will be in the dialysis field for years and years. A career is different from a job, and means that you love what you do and will be there for a long time. A job is basically a position you hold to pay the bills and keep food on the table, but you may not like going to that place to work. You may feel upset that you're working there long hours, and these feelings rub off on your coworkers and patients. If you've ever had a job instead of a career, you can relate to this feeling. However, in dialysis it is crucial to understand that days, months, and years go by super-fast, and you don't want to be stuck in a position that meets your needs at home but doesn't give you the ultimate excitement to come to work and be the best you can be. If you're seeking a career in dialysis, you'll put your whole heart into whatever you do and you won't be there to give cheap service to the patients.

Understand that just like any workplace you might have teammates with whom you don't always get along. You may be working for many years together, and you need to understand how to properly handle different situations that can arise. If you're reading this book and you've gotten the job but want out, please consider making goals and reaching them one step at a time—and being persistent in your own quest to get into something that you really love and appreciate.

Dialysis Schools & Certifications

A couple of dialysis schools are great and prep you well to become a hemodialysis technician—and they make sure you're state certified. And some schools only give you their own certificate stating that you are approved and are certified—only by them—to operate in a dialysis environment. This is totally different from being a state certified hemodialysis technician by a clinic or school.

There are two certifications you can test for and obtain. You don't have to get both; you can get one or the other. I know people who have both and I soon will have both, but I began and continued my career with just one. One is the Board of Nephrology Examiners Nursing and Technology (BONENT) certification, and the other is the Certified Clinical Hemodialysis Technician (CCHT) certification that comes from the Nephrology Nursing Certification Commission (NNCC). Having either of these certificates will get you any dialysis job because each state requires one or the other.

Schools like Star Academy are good in terms of making sure you're BONENT certified. The BONENT is awesome because they have various options to help you get certified quickly. Any dialysis school is good as long as they assist you in obtaining a job and getting certified once you complete their program.

In order to get the CCHT certificate and work in any of the fifty states, you have to work the last eighteen months in a dialysis unit for experience, and then you can take the CCHT certification test and pass it. Whatever dialysis school you look at, first ask how they will help you get a job, or are they accredited to certify you. Do this before you spend your money and the training is over. This is biggest disappointment for those who have graduated from a dialysis school—they can't find a job because they received no assistance or information in getting certified, and felt like they've wasted their money. A list of approved programs is at the end of this book.

Passing The Certification

Both the Board of Nephrology Examiners Nursing Technology (BONENT) and Nephrology Nursing Certification Commission (NNCC) allows you to choose several ways to complete the testing. You can choose paper and pencil or go to a computerized location in your district. Please visit their websites (listed at the end of this book) to participate in the mock test (consisting of 50 questions) if you need a head start on what to expect. The mock test isn't free and runs from thirty dollars and up. You can also read up on other resources on their website that can help you also. According to BONENT, in order to pass their testing you would need to get a 70 or above, anything less will disqualify you from receiving the certification. Their reporting scale ranges from 1 - 100. According to NNCC it clearly states below that the "CCHT exam contains 150 questions and must be completed in 180 minutes. A correct response rate of between 70 and 75% is required to pass the exam, depending on the version of the test".

Keeping Up That Certification

Depending on which certification you obtain, the process of staying certified differs slightly. The CCHT must be renewed every three years and requires submitting 30 credits from dialysis-related educational classes, or purchasing the recommended book materials, or even retaking the test. A minimum of 3000 hours of work experience as a hemodialysis technician within the three-year certification period is also required in order to apply for recertification.

The BONENT must be renewed every four years and requires submitting 40 contact hours of dialysis-related classes (online or offline, as long as there's proof you completed it), or you can retake the test, or apply for a waiver to excuse you from submitting credits.

Organization	BONENT	CCHT
Renewal	Renewed every 4 years.	Renew every 3 years.
Contact Hours	Requires 40 contact hours.	Require 30 contact hours.
Initial testing Prices	Computerized (250.00). Paper & Pencil (225.00).	Computerized (225.00).
Months allowed to get certified.	Allows 18 months upon being hired as a dialysis technician.	Allows 18 months upon being hired as a dialysis technician.
Recertify	1. Retesting. 2. Accumulate 40-contact hours. 3. One time waiver. Allows you to recertify without having to accumulate 40-contact hours. 4. To maintain a BONENT certification, nurses, technologists/technicians, and water specialists are required to pay an Annual Certification Fee of $60. 5. No fee to recertify but if your certification expired (13 months-10 years) it is 200.00 to renew and if the application is incomplete it is 65.00. If you choose to take the exam to renew you don't have to pay the 200.00 only the exam fee. 6. **BONENT states that you qualify for the 2021 Certification Amnesty Program** "if your Certification Expiration Date (as noted on your wallet card or in the BONENT database) is between January 1, 2011 and December 31, 2019."	1. Retesting. 2. The certificant must have at least 3,000 hours of work experience as a dialysis technician during within the three (3) years of the current certification period. 3. Anna offers a 6-month COVID-10 recertification grace period if you have been directly impacted by the pandemic. 4. Recertify by continuing education is 100.00. Recertify by exam is 225.00.
OTHER INFO	BONENT states "CMS will allow patient care technicians to continue working even if they have not achieved certification within 18 months of hire or have not met on time renewals."	CCHT states "If you have worked a minimum of 5 years and 5000 hours as a dialysis technician, you may be eligible to apply for the advanced CCHT-A examination."

Figure 1

For Experienced Technicians Who Resigned

If you have left the dialysis profession and it's been over a year since your certification license has expired, there is

10

hope for you to renew your certification and get back out there. If you have received a BONENT certification, you must submit 40 contact hours from the past four years and pay the $200 Expired Certification Fee. According to BONENT.com you will not qualify to use the one-time waiver that excuses you from doing nothing to recertify. If you have received your CCHT certificate and it has expired since you have been out of the dialysis profession, and it has been over a year. The Nephrology Nursing Certification Commission requires that you apply to take the certification examination again, meeting all current eligibility criteria listed on their website for certification to become certified again. If either company ever ask you to get your supervisor to sign anything, and you have been out of work for a long time, you must go back to your last supervisor at the job and ask them to signature it.

Preparing To Get Hired

In terms of filling a position, many clinical managers can sense if you're just looking at the money, or if you'll provide care without complaints from patients and your teammates about carelessness, bad attitude, and disregard for self-improvement. Many interested people often tell me how they've sent their resume to different dialysis clinics with no response.

You must think about how you'll present yourself for that job. I have friends who are clinical managers and they don't play around when it's time to hire. They look at everything and check you out. I repeat, things are tougher now than when I started. Many clinics now require you to upload your resume and apply online only, so find out. With online uploading, the manager can't put a personality to the resume. That's why I recommend going inside the clinic to drop off your resume, if possible. I've seen some ridiculously tall resume stacks, and they keep growing. This is a great time to seriously stand out. In this type of occupation, every company is paying above state minimum wage. I suggest you call first before going.

For example, call and say, "Hi, my name is X. I'd like to know the clinical manager's name and ask if he/she is available to briefly meet with me. I'd really like to drop off my resume in person." If you get transferred to the clinical manager and that person is rude on the phone, or nonchalant, please don't give up. Continue your quest to get a job in dialysis. Rudeness is the number one complaint I've been hearing lately, but don't let that to hold you back. Apply elsewhere. Just keep saying, "I will get this job."

If the clinical manager gives you the okay, then dress nicely, go inside the center, and introduce yourself to the unit clerk out front. Ask to hand your resume directly to the clinical manager. If the unit clerk says to leave it with him/her, then don't argue, just leave it. But, before you do, say, "I talked to the manager on the phone, and I want to present my best to him/her because this job is important to me. Is it possible for me to leave it with (clinical manager's name)?"

All clinical managers are really busy. They have a lot of paperwork to do, monthly quotas to reach, responsibility for the whole unit, and other duties. Honestly, no time is good for them because of their workload. Sometimes the best time is in the afternoon, when their bellies are full and they're most relaxed. After you find out what time they will be available for you to drop off the resume package, make your professional move.

Cover Letter/Resume Police

Your cover letter and resume should be tailored to reflect any experience you have in caring for the sick or elderly, any experience as a health aide, phlebotomist, or any job assisting the ill. If you don't have experience, even though you paid to go to a dialysis school, all managers still desire experienced individuals. They'll tell you, "Yes, I see you just graduated but do you have experience?" You can put down any experience you've had helping people, even if it's a sickly family member, and the duties you performed for them, if you've visited nursing homes, or if you've helped children with developmental disabilities.

You can also mention that you know how to set up a machine, cater to patients, and you're a fast learner, whether you went to dialysis school or learned on your own. Be sure your resume is free of errors. If you're confused as to how your resume looks, use Google to find some articles on how to make it look professional, or visit this great site called http://www.fiverr.com. Skilled, incredible people can fix, format, and professionalize your cover letter and resume for only five dollars. They did it for me. Now that's awesome, right?

Employers are looking to train newbies and shouldn't discriminate against you in any way. You may have to go out of your way to clinics farther from the city that may need employees. Those clinics are sometimes short of staff because not everyone wants to commute, or the starting pay might be extremely low, or they may not have union. Many times I hear of a few technicians who come through those farther-out clinics, and after they get experience and certification, they apply to a different facility that's closer, offers more benefits, and has a higher rate of pay.

Pass the Test

Some corporate clinics will send you out, as they did me, for paid training if they just hired you from the interview. Or some clinics will start you immediately shadowing someone. I'll talk about this in Chapter 3. However, for some dialysis companies, you MUST pass the computer (or classroom) setting, and it's no joke. I've seen people so sad that they didn't pass the hire test and couldn't get the actual job, even though the clinical manager hired them for potential employment. It's up to the clinical manager in some corporate facilities to approve you to be retested, and many times they don't. You MUST pass the test. If not, no job!

However, some units have other penalties for not passing, like additional time with a preceptor, retaking the class, and other things. The supervisor who hired me continued to remind me to study or she couldn't let me in, so please study. It was tough for me at first learning about machines, access arms, information about the water room (where the water is purified and dialysate components are mixed, and distributed throughout the dialysis unit) and state regulations. I almost didn't make it, but my supervisor constantly reminded me that if I didn't pass I couldn't work.

Those words playing in my head motivated me, plus the encouragement of an educator, Mr. Richard Davis, was key. I really respect my past educator because he told me to read things more slowly and rethink the answers before I put them down on paper. His encouragement was, "You can be the best in dialysis if you set your mind to it" and I feel that you too can be the best if you are serious about this profession. I'll always respect him for his help and extra encouragement, no matter what. If it wasn't for him prodding me in the right way, I wouldn't be writing this book today. If you graduate by passing the clinical tests, you'll work another few weeks or months on the floor with a preceptor (a technician or nurse assigned to help you so you're properly trained and experienced).

Within this period of time, you will be reminded, reprimanded, and trained to handle the dialysis environment, including emergencies, patient issues, electronic paperwork, opening and closing shifts, cannulation of accesses, initiating machine treatment, and hardest of all, turnover. Your awareness and ability to catch on is crucial, as this will shape your dialysis nature or "style" of work. After those months, you're on your own, but if you're stuck, please, please ask for help. 'I'll talk more about this later.

7 Reasons Why YOU Should Become a Hemodialysis Technician

1. The compensation can be very lucrative, depending on where you work.

2. You can work in any dialysis facility in the fifty states with either CCHT or BONENT.

3. You're helping to extend and save people's lives.

4. You have potential to grow and step up the ladder to become a nurse. (Some companies will reimburse you or pay for your schooling to become a registered nurse.)

5. Some companies have great health benefits, a pension, a 401k, and other fantastic perks.

6. Your schedule can be three workdays a week or less, depending on whether you're full time or part time.

7. You have the opportunity to become an expert team member and help others who are in training.

7 Reflections of an Unemployed Newbie

You haven't gotten anywhere yet but you want to be a dialysis technician, or maybe you just graduated from a dialysis school.

1. Start researching on how you can obtain your CPR certification so you can put that on your resume. You should tailor your resume and cover letter to reflect any experience you have working with a similar population.

2. Learn as much as you can about dialysis and speak and think positively. Submit your resume to all units, including those farther away, and don't give up.

3. Call the desired unit and find out if the clinical manager has time to receive your resume and cover letter.

4. If you receive approval to go in, dress your best and arrive at the unit on time.

5. Present yourself with a smile and, please, no street talking. Give your resume and cover letter to the clinical manager.

6. If you decide to go to school, please go to one that will state certify you at the end.

7. Get phlebotomy training just to keep your employment options open.

7 Reflections of a Hired Newbie

If you pass the clinical test and get the job, you:

1. Will be training with a preceptor.

2. May receive negative reaction from patients, who are skeptical of new employees because they fear you will put them on in a slow manner, waste time, or you won't know how to stick (insert a needle).

3. Will need time to cultivate a true professional style/learning the working style of your teammates.

4. Will have to take your time and exercise patience with patients who are sometimes rude or frightened.

5. Must juggle properly during turnover, which is taking off old shift patients and putting on the new shift.

6. May be the subject of gossip from staff and other personnel as "the new girl/guy."

7. Should be humble and take advice from the right people.

Frequently Asked Questions

I have phlebotomy certifications. Will they hire me?

Yes! Some clinical managers will hire you depending on what experience you present to them. All clinical managers are different and look for different things. All prefer someone with a degree, but if you show you are a hard worker and can learn fast, anything is possible.

I have no experience. Can I be a dialysis technician?

I started from nowhere. It all depends on the clinical manager hiring you.

Clinical managers continue to tell me they want experienced technicians and that I can't apply because I'm not experienced. What should I do?

You can always apply and, depending on the clinical manager, they can still hire you with no experience and train you their way so you can become experienced. But It's best if you apply when you see an open position rather than assume a particular company is hiring when they're not.

A clinical manager was rude when I called/dropped off my resume. Should I follow up on the job?

Continue dropping off resumes and being friendly, because you just might be called back. Keep trying other centers.

I have experience but can't get a job in dialysis! What else should I do?

You should definitely research if a company has a union or not, and try to find out how to apply through their union.

Try to get hired into a staffing agency that gives bonuses and higher rates. Google "dialysis staffing agencies."

I went to dialysis school but can't get a job. What can I try?

Some schools don't offer BONENT exam certifications, and a dialysis school certificate only certifies that you have passed their required test showing that you know the different components of dialysis, and various aspects of the dialysis world. This is different from obtaining a certificate from a qualified company showing you passed the BONENT test. If you get into a school that will certify you, say that in your resume. Just continue to put your resume out there and be positive.

I've filled out so many applications. I just came out of dialysis school. It's been months and no one has called me back! I'm frustrated! What advice do you have?

Have you tried private clinics or clinics that are farther away? Those clinics need the most help. Continue to read this book to discover how to overcome these obstacles and how to present yourself.

I got the job but it's not how you described it. In some instances, it's tougher than I expected! Should I just give up?

Again, this is only my experience. I'm not going to lie. It is tough, but you can do it. Give it a chance before considering a change.

I went to a BONENT-approved program and want to know if I can begin working on the floor after I'm hired?

It depends on which company hires you. If it's corporate, you'll be sent for retraining on their company's policies and procedures.

CHAPTER #2
SIMPLE BASICS & CLINICAL LANGUAGE

The brain doesn't say learning is hard, your feelings do.

This chapter elaborates on a few basic definitions you should understand before you hit an interview. They'll help you know what's being talked about and enable you to understand the clinical manager and the job demands better. Please study all you can about dialysis by researching online, especially if you've never gone to dialysis school. Some books give you a thorough breakdown on every definition, like the Review of Hemodialysis for Nurses and Dialysis Personnel. Books and video demonstrations are also excellent if you're studying to pass the certification exam. I mention more dialysis-related books and educational materials at the end of this book. In the meantime, I'll run through a few important definitions you should understand concerning dialysis.

A Few Basics

Acute Kidney Disease- Acute kidney failure (AKF) occurs when the kidneys suddenly become unable to filter waste products from the blood. When the kidneys lose their filtering ability, dangerous levels of wastes may accumulate and the blood's chemical makeup may get out of balance.

21

Chronic Kidney Disease- Chronic kidney disease (CKD) is defined as damaged kidneys, or a reduction in kidney function below 60 percent of normal. Kidney disease is sometimes called a "silent" disease, because it often causes no pain or other symptoms.

Test Used to show if one has Kidney disease

Urinalysis- a test that checks a sample of urine for the amount of protein, blood (red blood cells and white blood cells) and other things. Protein and red and white blood cells are not normally found in the urine, so having too much of any of these may mean kidney disease.

Glomerular filtration rate (GFR). GFR is estimated from results of a serum (or blood) creatinine test. The GFR tells how well the kidneys are working to remove wastes from the blood. It is the best way to check kidney function.

Dialysis- Dialysis is the procedure for artificially replacing many functions performed by normal kidneys. It is necessary to replace kidney function when kidneys are no longer able to keep people healthy and safe. There are two common types of dialysis: hemodialysis (in-center treatment) and peritoneal dialysis.

Peritoneal Dialysis- is another way to remove waste products from the blood when the kidneys can no longer do the job adequately. During peritoneal dialysis, blood vessels in the abdominal lining (peritoneum) fill in for the kidneys, with the help of a fluid (dialysate) that flows into and out of the peritoneal space. Peritoneal dialysis differs from hemodialysis, because it is usually done at home and doesn't require filtering the patient's blood to clean out the toxins.

In-Center Hemodialysis- Patients come 3 times a week in the daytime to complete treatment in a series of 3-4 hours, on a dialysis machine. In hemodialysis, a dialysis machine and a special filter called an artificial kidney, or a dialyzer, are used to clean the blood.

In-center nocturnal hemodialysis- Some companies offer nighttime dialysis treatments. Meaning the patient would come to treatment 3 or 4 times a week in the nighttime and complete treatment, the pace of treatment would be slowed to 6-8 hours. The nocturnal dialysis treatment is usually slower and for a longer period of time. This means the treatment is gentler for the body to tolerate, while removing a greater amount of wastes and fluid from the blood. The blood is much "cleaner" and blood tests will be better.

PPE - Personal Protective Equipment (gloves, shield, apron or gown, face mask, or goggles). Super important—always wear it. Some units will terminate you if you're caught cannulating without them.

Your Machine - Models such as the K2, T machine, or others, depending on which unit hires you; not all companies use the same machine. (Watch videos on priming different machines and setting up dialyzers.) Some machines also have electronic charts inside them.

Extracorporeal Circuit - The blood pump system/lines used to set up the machine.

Dialyzers - This is the whole purpose of hemodialysis, which is to use this artificial kidney to filter out blood toxins, which the kidneys can no longer do. (Depending on the center, the dialyzer shape/size could be different.)

Normal Saline Bag - The 0.9% saline solution you'll use to prime the dialyzer and to make the extracorporeal circuit soluble for cleaning the blood. Saline can be used to give medications, as a rinse back after treatment, and for flushes to help prevent clots from forming in the extracorporeal circuit for patients who aren't on anticoagulants.

Bicarbonate/Acid Ports - Solutions created in the water room to clean the blood. The acid can also be prescription bottles sealed or put into jugs for individual patients.

Water Room- This is where the bicarbonate and acid is created, mixed and distributed to the dialysis machines on the floor. The Reverse Osmosis (RO) is also located in this room with a host of other water purification machines and storage tanks.

BFR (Blood Flow Rate), DFR (Dialysis Flow Rate), BVP (Blood Volume Processed through the dialyzer) Kt/V and URR (measures of your delivered dose of dialysis. They tell whether you are receiving the right amount of dialysis.) - Study the different results of the above definitions, because it's what you'd be putting in the electronic flow sheets at the end of treatment. I've seen clinics that don't set their machines to give these results and go by other standards, such as monthly blood work, so be aware of that.

CRIT-LINE® III - Some hospitals and centers use this computer system that connects to the dialyzer and is designed to challenge the patient to remove appropriate fluid, and prevent the patient from cramping (crashing) on the machine.

pHoenix Dialysate Meter - Can be used to test the conductivity of bicarbonate mixed in the water room, and to compare results to the dialysis machine. This meter also has other helpful uses in testing the PH of water in various instances.

Computer - Monitoring individual patients using electronic charting paper system, or some units will still use old-fashioned charting, which means monitoring patients using a pen and paper. Some units have the computer inside the machine. Every center has a desktop.

Cannulation - The act of inserting a needle into the patient's fistula or graft access for treatment. Additional definition information is in Chapter 5.

Ladder Rope Technique- The rope ladder technique rotates the needle placement sites each time the patient has hemodialysis. The new needle site should be about one-and-a-half to two inches from the last puncture site.

Button Hole Method- The buttonhole technique is a way to "cannulate," which means "to insert dialysis needles." Instead of sharp, pointed needles, dull needles are placed into the exact same holes on the fistula every time the patient undergoes dialysis. After around 10 cannulations using the sharp dialysis needles, the buttonhole site will develop a scar tunnel track. This track is the similar as a pierced ear that has scar tissue formed and will cause less to no pain and bleeding when cannulating. After the buttonhole is created, a blunt dialysis needle is used, which eliminates the risks of cuts and bleeding to the tract.

Needles - 14, 15, 16, 17 needles or, 15 and 14 white needles are the biggest needles I've seen, and run on a blood flow up to 500-550; 17 needles are the smallest for brand-new accesses, depending on the doctor's order. Depending on which company you work for, the needles come in different shapes and sizes.

Infiltrated- When the needle punctures both walls of the access, blood leaks into the tissues and causes swelling, and often a painful bruise. The escaped blood can compress the access. This may cause stenosis (narrowing of the blood vessel) and/or a blood clot that could damage the access— or even cause it to fail.

Main medications - Ask the nurse at your unit to explain which iron, anticoagulant, and other meds are being used, because a medication can sometimes be recalled and a new one replaces it. Some dialysis units frequently change policy, procedures, medications, and protocols. Also, some units in different states allow their hemodialysis technicians to give anticoagulants. Please check with your clinic and understand that no two states' regulations are the same. Many states allow only the RN to give anticoagulants, so be sure—this is important.

Clinical Language

Having cramps/crashing

Patients experience this while on the machine. This can be due to the rapid fluid and electrolyte shifts in and out of muscle cells from the hemodialysis treatment (or you are pulling too much fluid off by setting the goal of fluid too high, or the patient needs a change of dry weight). The patient could be cramping for many reasons, but first things first: Follow your clinic's policy to stop the cramping.

Can I have a double?

Meaning can you or another teammate provide a second signature on the electronic computer to show that you properly used the pHoenix meter, and tested the machine so treatment can begin. This depends on the unit you work for, as all charting systems are different.

Did you make some packs?

Meaning did you create a bundle of a few supplies needed for pre- and posttreatment to use on the patient. In Chapter 7, farther on, you'll see what I mean.

A chuck

A blue lightweight pad used to put supplies on for patients pre- and post-treatment. It is also placed under the patient's arm to prevent any blood from getting on their clothes.

Can you open and close the unit?

Meaning can you open the unit early in the morning, before 5:00 a.m., set up the machines, and hold down the water room. Closing is when you stay behind and make sure all the dialysis machines are shut down properly and the water room is taken care of properly. The responsibility differs depending on the responsibilities given for being a closer.

Brief Description of Your Main Team Members

Medical Doctors - Deal with patients' overall health progress and some doctors cover the whole unit's operations.

Clinical Managers - Supervise overall unit progress/patient complaints/staff relations. Many come to work at 9:00 a.m. or 10:00 a.m., but they usually create their own start time.

Charge Nurse - Makes sure issues on the treatment floor are handled appropriately and the flow of treatment dialysis is safe and in order.

Nurses - Initiate treatment in many states for catheters, prepare medications, and other various duties on the floor.

Social Workers - Deal with some medical insurance issues, as well as human resources for dialysis patients and much more.

Dietician -Deals with proper eating habits/explaining results of blood work and other duties.

Unit clerks - Front desk workers who deal with transportation and other important paperwork and duties.

Administrative Assistants - Assist clinical managers, charge nurses, and staff, and deal with payroll issues and other vast duties.

Educators - If your unit has them, they usually come on the floor often to make sure the staff is updated on new clinical protocols and proper procedures.

Other teammates - Dialysis assistants, equipment technicians, computer technicians, blood-work drivers, ambulance drivers, and housekeepers.

More Frequently Asked Questions

-What if I don't understand how to prime?

Research priming, search videos, and if possible, stop by a dialysis school for information.

-How do I get the air out of the dialyzer?

It's difficult to explain in writing because it's nothing like doing it practically, I suggest you speak to your trainer (preceptor).

-Will my preceptor still help me when I'm on my own?

Yes, they should assist you with any questions, situations, or worries.

-What are the reasons I could be fired?

There are many. A few I've seen are a technician having an outburst on the floor, unprofessional behavior, detrimental situations, fraud (incorrect information put in for the patient), and improper monitoring of patients, forgetting to sign off on your important assigned duties.

-Can I give some medications?

Depending on your state's clinical protocols, some states allow technicians to give medications, such as heparin.

-If the nurse pressures me to give medications, what should I do?

Never do it! You don't want anyone, especially the patient, to accuse you of breaking rules. I've seen it happen.

-Can I give Normal Saline?

In some instances, some states consider this a medication while the patient is on the machine. This is different from using it to prime the machine. Please find out.

-How much saline can I prime with or give to the patient?

Again, it depends on the unit you're hired into. Each unit has different protocols.

CHAPTER #3
HEMODIALYSIS T MACHINE
SETUP & INFO

Fight procrastination and win.

There are three machine types that I am familiar with, the H, K, and T in-center hemodialysis machines & this method of priming can be used on all three machines. I will only talk about how to set-up a regular T machine. Now, there are two types of T machines, one is a regular T machine and the other is a BlueStar® T machine. Both T machines have a chairside interface built into them which makes it easier to access information about the patient. The regular T machine is more time-consuming with priming & set-up whereas the BlueStar® T will test the machine while you set it up. You connect the transducers, Hansens, put the venous chamber line in the air detector, and then press "auto prime" and the machine does the work. If you will be in a unit that doesn't utilize the K, or T machine please use YouTube and Google to get the information you need on setup.

What supplies do I need?

You need a bag of normal saline, the prescribed dialyzer, and the extracorporeal circuit known as bloodlines. Please inspect all items for defects and look for the expiration dates. You also need to make sure that the prescribed dialyzer doesn't have any cracks or discoloration.

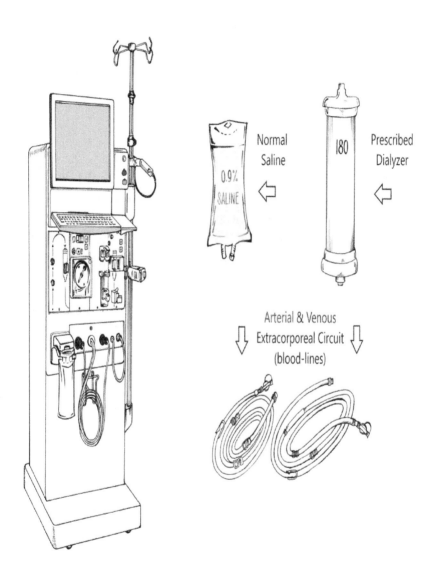

Normal
Saline

Prescribed
Dialyzer

Arterial & Venous
Extracorporeal Circuit
(blood-lines)

STEP #1

Ensure the dialysis machine is clean and has no blood spots. Once the machine is clean, open the saline bag and hang it on the IV pole, and put the prescribed dialyzer in the holder. Open the blood lines & hold the arterial line in your left hand and the venous line in your right hand.

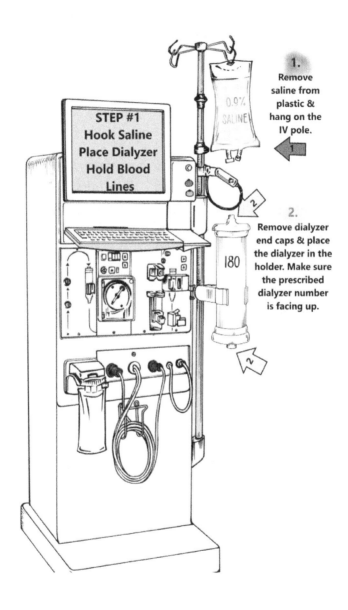

STEP #1
Hook Saline
Place Dialyzer
Hold Blood
Lines

1.
Remove saline from plastic & hang on the IV pole.

2.
Remove dialyzer end caps & place the dialyzer in the holder. Make sure the prescribed dialyzer number is facing up.

STEP #2

Set-up the arterial line.

Set-up the arterial lines on the machines and connect the flat end to the top of the dialyzer. You need to make sure that your saline line, transducer, heparin line, and medicine line are clamped. Now, connect the arterial saline line to the saline bag that's on the IV.

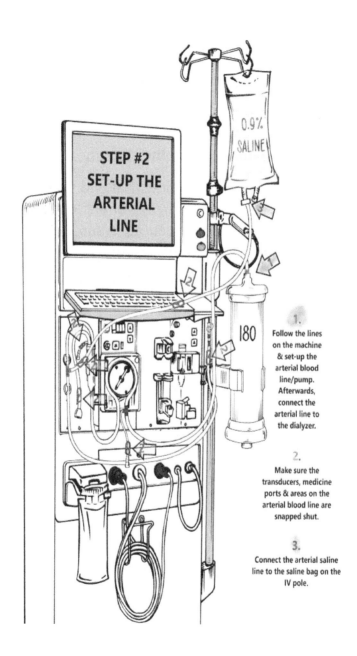

**STEP #2
SET-UP THE
ARTERIAL
LINE**

0.9%
SALINE

1.
Follow the lines
on the machine
& set-up the
arterial blood
line/pump.
Afterwards,
connect the
arterial line to
the dialyzer.

2.
Make sure the
transducers, medicine
ports & areas on the
arterial blood line are
snapped shut.

3.
Connect the arterial saline
line to the saline bag on the
IV pole.

STEP #3

Set-up the venous lines on the machine.

Proceed to connect the venous flat end to the bottom of the dialyzer and place the patient venous end on the dialyzer holder. Make sure your venous transducer and medicine port is clamped shut. Don't clamp the venous patient end just yet.

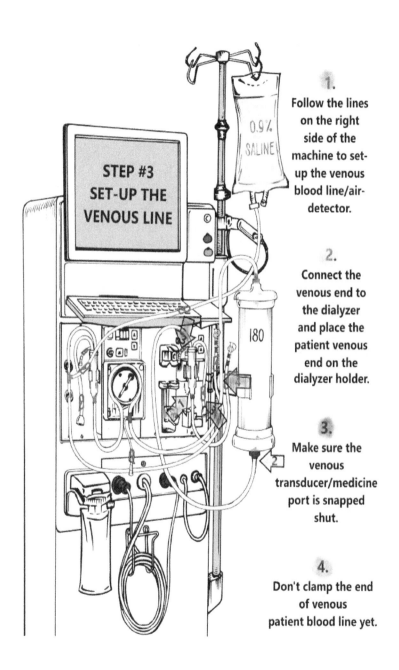

**STEP #3
SET-UP THE
VENOUS LINE**

1. Follow the lines on the right side of the machine to set-up the venous blood line/air-detector.

2. Connect the venous end to the dialyzer and place the patient venous end on the dialyzer holder.

3. Make sure the venous transducer/medicine port is snapped shut.

4. Don't clamp the end of venous patient blood line yet.

STEP #4

Prime the patient end arterial line.

Take the patient end arterial & venous lines from the dialyzer holder and place them in the white bucket that is on the side of the machine. Unclamp the patient arterial end and the saline line. Now allow saline to run out of the arterial patient end. Once the air is gone, proceed to clamp the arterial patient end.

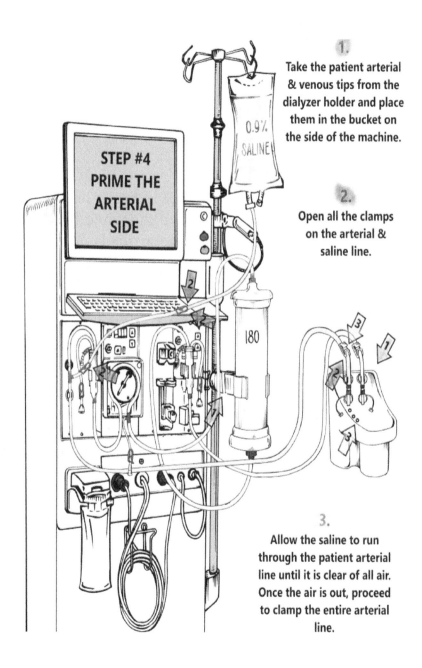

STEP #4
PRIME THE
ARTERIAL
SIDE

0.9%
SALINE

180

1. Take the patient arterial
& venous tips from the
dialyzer holder and place
them in the bucket on
the side of the machine.

2. Open all the clamps
on the arterial &
saline line.

3. Allow the saline to run
through the patient arterial
line until it is clear of all air.
Once the air is out, proceed
to clamp the entire arterial
line.

STEP #5

Prime the rest of the arterial side.

Take the patient end arterial & venous lines from the dialyzer holder and place them in the white bucket that is on the side of the machine. Now, unclamp the patient arterial end and the arterial saline line. Now, let the saline flow out of the patient's end of the arterial line. After the air is gone, clamp the patient's arterial end port. You will leave the arterial patient's end that you just primed in the bucket and turn your focus to priming the rest of the circuit. You will now open the small medicine port that is by the transducer and fill the arterial chamber to the level listed on the machine with saline. You are doing this to prevent more air from going into the blood pump and into the dialyzer. Once you have done this, you will now turn-on the blood pump and raise it to 150.

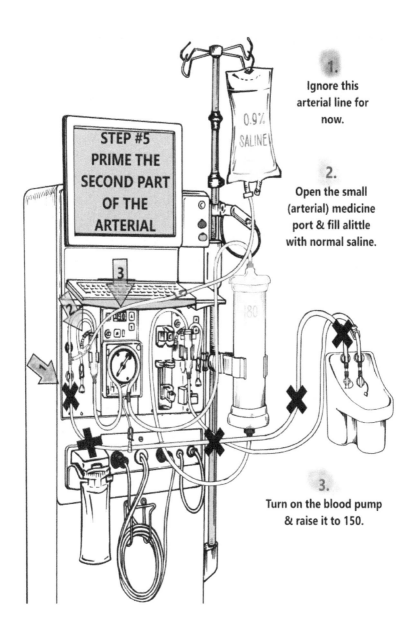

**STEP #5
PRIME THE
SECOND PART
OF THE
ARTERIAL**

0.9%
SALINE

1. Ignore this arterial line for now.

2. Open the small (arterial) medicine port & fill alittle with normal saline.

3. Turn on the blood pump & raise it to 150.

43

STEP #6

Prime the venous line/flip the dialyzer.

You will begin to see the saline trickle into the venous chamber and out through the patient venous end that is in the bucket. At this point, you need to turn the dialyzer upside down (venous end up). You will see the air bubbles that have gathered at the top of the dialyzer. Now, lightly tap the dialyzer to make sure all of the air comes out.

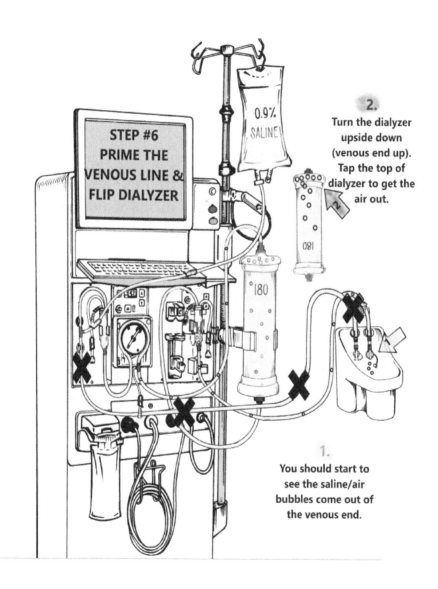

STEP #6
PRIME THE
VENOUS LINE &
FLIP DIALYZER

2. Turn the dialyzer upside down (venous end up). Tap the top of dialyzer to get the air out.

1. You should start to see the saline/air bubbles come out of the venous end.

STEP #7

Test the machine.

Now that the arterial and venous is primed, it is now time to test the machine. You will first stop the blood pump and clamp the venous end which is in the white bucket. The arterial should already be clamped. You will then connect the arterial and venous ends, open the clamps and hang them on the IV pole. Turn the dialyzer back to arterial (red) side up. Start the blood pump and let it run a little before testing. Find the test interface on the machine and press "both" tests. If the machine fails any of those tests try your best to troubleshoot the problem or call the equipment technician.

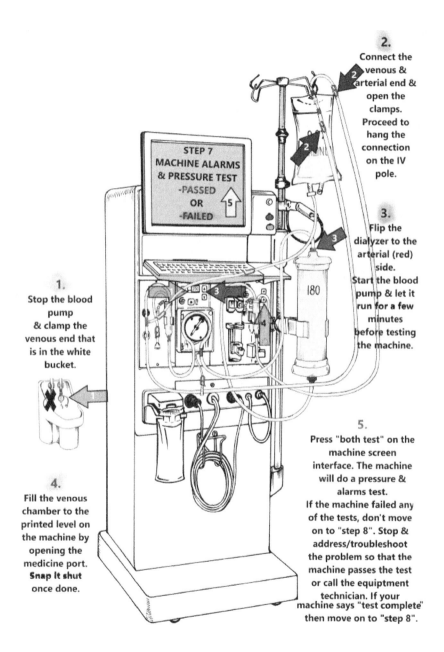

2.
Connect the venous & arterial end & open the clamps. Proceed to hang the connection on the IV pole.

STEP 7 MACHINE ALARMS & PRESSURE TEST -PASSED OR -FAILED

3.
Flip the dialyzer to the arterial (red) side. Start the blood pump & let it run for a few minutes before testing the machine.

1.
Stop the blood pump & clamp the venous end that is in the white bucket.

4.
Fill the venous chamber to the printed level on the machine by opening the medicine port. **Snap It shut** once done.

5.
Press "both test" on the machine screen interface. The machine will do a pressure & alarms test. If the machine failed any of the tests, don't move on to "step 8". Stop & address/troubleshoot the problem so that the machine passes the test or call the equiptment technician. If your machine says "test complete" then move on to "step 8".

STEP #8

Connect & Recirculate.

Connect Hansens & recirculate.

Attach the arterial & venous transducers to the machine. Plug your red Hansen to the arterial side of the dialyzer and the blue Hansen to the venous side. Place the venous chamber into the air detector and allow the set-up to recirculate.

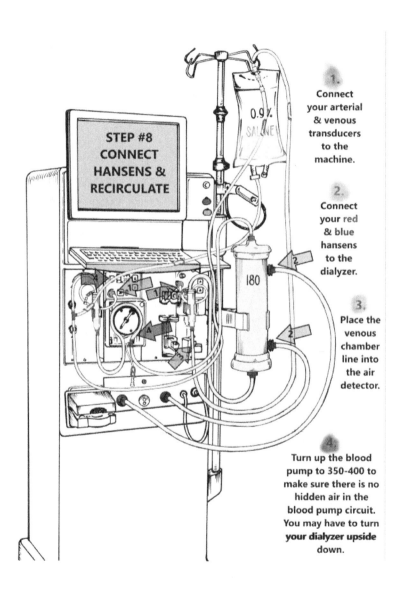

STEP #8
CONNECT
HANSENS &
RECIRCULATE

0.9%
SALINE

180

1. Connect your arterial & venous transducers to the machine.

2. Connect your red & blue hansens to the dialyzer.

3. Place the venous chamber line into the air detector.

4. Turn up the blood pump to 350-400 to make sure there is no hidden air in the blood pump circuit. You may have to turn **your dialyzer upside** down.

49

SET-UP COMPLETE

The machine is now ready for a patient.

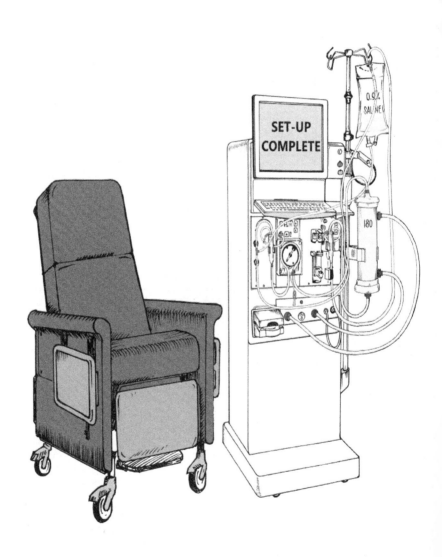

CHAPTER #4
TRAINING WITH YOUR PRECEPTOR

Your gift can make room for you if you are meek and humble.

Once you've landed the job or passed the required test, your next step is to train with a certified staff member, such as a Patient Care Technician Preceptor, a qualified individual who's good at showing newbies the ropes of the position. He/She should make sure the newcomer learns everything correctly, according to the company's protocol. You'll be learning so much in this stage of hemodialysis. That's why it's crucial that the right preceptor is overseeing you. If not, you'll be taught incorrectly and it will show when you're finished with the training stage and you're out on the floor serving patients without the assistance of a preceptor. I've had a few preceptors due to different circumstances. I considered myself a floater, shadowing different individuals, but I did pick it up rather quickly. In a matter of three to four months, I was on the floor doing my thing.

Initially, I didn't have a good way of dealing with the normal patient backlash. Patients tend to criticize and instruct, and I felt bad when I didn't know how to deal with them right away. But other than that, I felt that I was a great technician. I really worked hard and patients began to love me. I remember one awesome preceptor, J Jackson, who was once a dialysis assistant like me, and later became a dialysis technician. Now she's a dialysis teacher in New York. I definitely won't forget her and will always appreciate her excellence in showing me the ins and outs of the job of dialysis assistant. When I became a technician, she was there again to show me the way. She was a great example of a preceptor; she was very friendly to patients and to her teammates—and she showed me the correct way to care for patients.

She was really good at solving issues among personnel in the unit. I was the type to hold in stuff and not appropriately express what I was feeling to those I felt were causing problems. After a year of gaining experience, after a year of training, a charge nurse wanted me to retrain with a different preceptor. No patients had complained about me, only the charge nurse; but eventually everything cooled down and I came out on top again. No hard feelings anymore. I've learned a lot about what makes a professional preceptor. That situation is buried and I'm moving forward. I will now list the characteristics that indicate whether you have a professional preceptor or a nonprofessional preceptor; plus, what to look out for when it comes to the patients, and much more.

7 Characteristics of a Professional Preceptor

1. Will give you clinical protocols.

2. Will understand this is a learning stage and not overly ridicule or loudly make fun of you.

3. Will be patient and understanding.

4. Will have great patient care skills.

5. Will show you how to be a team player.

6. Will encourage you at all times.

7. Will not gossip about your mistakes to other employees.

7 Characteristics of an Unprofessional Preceptor

1. Will take advantage of you by letting you do all his/her work, clean all their patients' messes, and call it learning instead of working together.

2. Will be very rude and seem to not want you shadowing them, treating you as if you're a bother.

3. Will show you nothing but crazy shortcuts instead of clinical protocols.

4. Will have zero patient care skills, be rude and disrespectful to patients, and have an attitude problem.

5. Will complain and gossip about other teammates and will want you to take sides, or will complain to them about you being new.

6. Will not teach you how to prepare anything during your downtime, and is just plain lazy or nasty.

7. Will be flirty and make inappropriate advances instead of showing you how to do the work.

If you have a good teacher, that's excellent, but if you have a poor preceptor you should talk to your clinical manager or educator in private and share your feelings, backed up by documentation. You shouldn't back off from telling the truth for fear of hurting someone. Keep in mind that your job is on the line, and you're dealing with human beings in life-or-death situations here. One simple, bad mistake can cost a life —and create a negative ripple effect.

For the sake of anyone depending on you, be sure you're trained properly, according to the policies of your unit. If someone tells you this unprofessional preceptor is the only person you can shadow, don't get an attitude with that preceptor. Just continue studying books about proper procedures according to your clinical protocols.

More things you will learn

1. Needle Stick Safety.

2. Isolation room procedures.

3. How to draw blood work and store bloods taken.

4. Documentation (clinical variance, charts.)

5. Health Insurance Portability and Accountability Act (HIPPA) laws and State Regulations.

6. Personal Private Information regulations.

7. Professionalism.

8. Drug test policies.

9. Handling resuscitations and on the floor emergencies.
10. Proper Teamwork.

CHAPTER #5
REAL PATIENT ASSESSMENT&
COMMON PRETREATMENT
COMPLICATIONS

Air can be your best friend and your worst enemy.

Now that you are on the floor training, you will be taught how to handle patients who are new admissions, transients (from other units), elderly, middle-aged, and young. In any case, I encourage you to first greet your patients and assess whether they may be blind, deaf, or using a cane or a wheelchair to assist them. Remove their heavy purses, bags, and outerwear (coats, jackets, heavy sweaters, and boots), then weigh each patient, escort each to their chair, and ask the following:

-How are you feeling? Dizzy? Short of breath (SOB)? Fever? Chills?

-Have you been admitted to the hospital since your last treatment? If yes, do you have the discharge papers to give the nurse?

If all is well, proceed according to either your unit's protocols or a suggested three-step cannulation method mentioned later in this book. If the patient needs oxygen, please put on the blood pressure cuff and call the nurse to evaluate that patient. If the nurse gives the ok then get the oxygen machine with cannula and ask how much oxygen to give only if you are authorized to give it. Many states view oxygen as a nurse's duty or a medication order.

Below I list a few reasons for common complications in dialysis.

Some Reasons for Shortness of Breath

-Fluid overload.

-Maybe a recent surgery/operation.

-Other recently developed health issues.

Some Reasons for Fever/Chills

-Infection/sepsis.

If a patient comes in and the temperature is high, if the patient complains of serious chills, and if you see the patient is cold, clammy, and sweating, notify the nurse ASAP before starting any treatment. The nurse may be able to get the doctor to grant permission for special blood work and antibiotics to be given to that patient while on treatment. Many times, patients who experience chills and a fever have gotten an infection in their blood called sepsis. Signs of sepsis often include shivering uncontrollably, and saying it's cold when, indeed, the room temperature is normal and other patients aren't complaining.

Being savvy regarding complications is a huge plus, because you can save the patient's life faster when you know what you're doing and why you're doing it. I've listed a few complications below, and I want you to find out how your unit handles each one. If you don't have the job yet, research online how to handle these situations so you can explain, if asked by the manager, what you would do in any of these instances. This will show that you're familiar with complications and can learn how to handle them according to unit protocol. I'm telling you, this is so important to know.

Complications

-Passing out.

-Cardiac arrest.

-Totally unresponsive.

-Seizures.

-Air in machine.

-Bleeding profusely while on machine.

Emergency Wisdom

I've dealt with patients with some of these treatment issues, and it requires my total concentration and knowledge on how to get things back to normal for the patient while they're undergoing treatment. I've witnessed patients go into cardiac arrest/seizures, become unresponsive, or pass out; and my first response was to initiate the emergency protocols I'd learned. If the patient becomes responsive but refuses to go to the hospital, you should document it. Also, the RN should do a clinical variance report and any other required paperwork for the refusal.

Air Can = Death

When it comes to air in the extracorporeal circuit and dialyzer, all newbies should fully understand how to prime the dialyzer correctly. Incorrect priming is the number one reason for air getting into the venous chamber of the extracorporeal system in the first place. Some clinics say take out the blood pump part of the extracorporeal circuit first and elevate it up in a horizontal position so that the gravity can pull the air pocket out of the blood pump before you begin priming. Sometimes even though you prime correctly, there are other ways that air can get into the system. One reason is forgetting to completely clamp the saline line. Once this happens all of the saline goes into the blood pump system and then enters the patient then when the saline bag is empty air begins to travel through the extracorporeal circuit and dialyzer.

Thankfully the venous part of the machine has an air detector alarm. This will alarm staff that they need to do something ASAP to prevent any air gathered in the venous chamber of the machine from getting to the patient. Really learn how to get the air out of the system—and understand that the patients can die from air in their blood received from the venous air chamber of the machine. This is called an air embolism (air in their blood). Go over the unit protocol for assisting a patient who has developed air embolism symptoms.

Honestly, in all my years I've never seen a patient get an air embolism from a machine, and I'm thankful I've never witnessed it. Every unit has different protocols in terms of getting air out of the system. I'll list below what I've seen and heard.

- In some units, someone will bring a syringe, insert it into the venous port, and pull all the air out of the dialyzer in the air detector.

- In a few units, the policy is to discard everything and put up a new system if the air is severe.

Bleeding

I have witnessed patients' needle sites begin to bleed while on the machine, not a lot, but trickling down the arm from the site, either venous or arterial, or sometimes both. I clean up the blood completely and change the tape because I hate when blood saturates the tape. I like the patient to have a clean access at all times. Be a clean technician—you'll become known for it. I've dealt with a patient who started bleeding profusely after cannulation. I pulled the needle, notified the nurse, and recannulated after the bleeding stopped. Many units use peroxide and betadine because both are very good at reducing the bleeding, but always know the protocols before using them.

Notifying the Nurse

I got into a lot of trouble in my younger days for not notifying the nurse appropriately. Many times I worked with excellent, helpful, loving nurses; I also worked with rude, stubborn, and sometimes lazy nurses who blamed me for a lot, like forgetting to remind THEM to give the patients different meds, which I didn't feel was my duty. However, no matter what unfortunate situation you encounter, if that nurse is supervising your section that day, always notify him/her if you come up with unusual findings regarding the patients. Just be aware of every possible situation and don't give anyone a reason to write you up for a violation. Please, I repeat. Notify the nurse of any patient issues and document it if that nurse won't hear you out. Tell another nurse, or if it's really a severe problem, explain the situation to the clinical manager.

If an RN or teammate wants you to do anything against company policy, like putting in incorrect blood pressure, temperature, or other information, please document the truth! This is serious. Remember, these patients may have family and friends depending on them. Unfortunately, I've encountered unscrupulous personnel in many units. Do the right thing at all times and put the patient first. In addition, document in the computer that patient X had high blood pressure and nurse Y was notified.

If that patient leaves the unit then passes away, or something else detrimental happens, an investigation into what happened begins and will be traced back to the dialysis unit. Trust me; you can't lie, because you'll be exposed as crooked and deceitful.

Nonfiction Crooked Situations

Scenario #1 – You're in charge of Mr. X's treatment on Tuesday. Toward the end of his treatment he tells you he feels sick. You take his temperature and it's 100° in both ears. You tell the nurse. The nurse goes to him and asks him in what way he feels sick. He says his stomach. She tells him, "Oh, take it easy. You'll feel better. Okay, hon?" You tell the nurse you want to document the incident, and she says no. On top of that, she changes the temperature to 97°. So Mr. X goes home, his body temperature rises to 106° degrees, and he goes to the emergency room. He misses his treatment at your facility on Thursday and Saturday due to being in the hospital. The following week you hear that he died due to a severe infection in his blood. This could've been prevented if blood cultures had been taken, and the doctor had been notified. So now an investigation is launched on why that patient died and what could've been done to prevent his death. It will be traced back to how he was feeling after treatment. What do you think about something like this? Would you continue to lie and say he was feeling all right or would you tell the truth?

Scenario #2 - You work with an unprofessional technician who doesn't monitor his patients appropriately, even dozing off in his section. You notice this behavior continue but you're afraid to confront the tech nicely about it, so it gets worse. One day Mr. Unprofessional has a new admission, a sickly, elderly patient who depends on frequent monitoring due to extreme low blood pressure and seizure episodes. This technician skips a session of monitoring this patient and the patient passes out. The tech calls for help and the team calls 911. This patient winds up in the hospital again, all due to not being monitored properly. What do you think about this and what would you do?

Scenario #3 - A nurse constantly tells a teammate of yours to push medications for her patients. She tells the technician she'll draw the meds and all the technician needs to do is push the medication. One day you see the technician draw up some of the medications and push them. You witness the patient passing out after receiving the meds, and that technician confesses she gave the wrong medicine. The nurse tells her, "Oh, I'll take the blame. Just say it was me." What do you think about this and what would you do?

10 Reflection Wisdom Tips

1. Don't ignore the slightest symptom of a complication. You could save a life by detecting it quickly.

2. Don't ignore blood slowly trickling down a patient's arm from the needle insertion sites by covering/patching it up with gauze or other materials. Get to the source of the bleeding and clean it.

3. Learn as much as you can about air. It's your best friend in life, but it can be your worst enemy in hemodialysis.

4. Learn as much as you can about CPR and know which patients don't want to be resuscitated (brought back to consciousness).

5. Don't be a jerky cannulator. When you stick, stretch the skin and insert the needle slowly and gently.

6. If someone in the unit is trembling and says they're extremely cold, and no one else is complaining about the temperature, you really should take their temperature.

7. No one is exempt from a patient bleeding profusely. It could be too much heparin or a stenosis in the vessel of the access. Learn about these causes.

8. Unprofessional nurses aren't discovered easily; it's usually the technician who's covering for them.

9. If you're an intelligent technician, protect yourself at all times through documentation. It will save you.

10. You shouldn't be serious buddies with anyone in the unit who might come before the duties of your job.

CHAPTER #6
LIFELINE ACCESS &
CANNULATION COMPLICATIONS

You're a complication watcher. The more you keep your eyes open, the quicker you can save a life.

In this chapter I will briefly explain the different accesses used to do hemodialysis, and relate a basic three-step cannulation method. Again, I stress this—please follow your clinical policy because these are merely my suggestions and every unit is different. Many types of lifelines are implanted into individuals, but I will speak only about the common ones and briefly explain their functions.

Lifelines (See Figure 2 on the following page)

Fistula(ae) - A fistula used for hemodialysis is a direct connection of an artery to a vein. Fistulas are created using your body's natural arteries and veins, which are amazing. This is the preferred type of access because, once the fistula properly matures and gets bigger and stronger; it provides access with good blood flow that can last for years and years.

Graft - A graft, an access made by using a piece of soft tube to join an artery and vein in your arm. A graft can be implanted in the neck, arm, wrist, or leg if the surgeon sees either that a patient has very small veins or that he can't create a fistula connection with the vein and artery.

Catheter - A soft tube that is placed in a large vein, usually in your neck. For dialysis, a catheter is sometimes located on the patient's neck, chest, or leg. A catheter is usually a short-term option; however, in some cases a catheter is used as a permanent access.

Types of Access for Dialysis

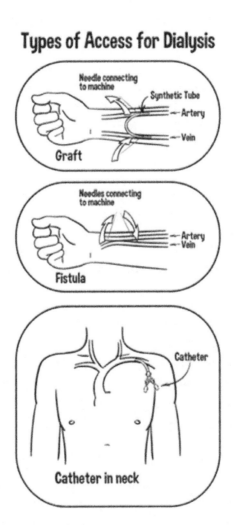

Figure 2

Three-Step Cannulation

Step 1 - Evaluate

If the patient has a catheter then the nurse usually connects them to the machine, depending on which state you're employed in. If your patient has a fistula or a graft, once the patient is seated you should look at their access, observe, and feel. It's called "feel the thrill" (the vibration of the pumping of blood in the access) and "hear the bruit" (the sound of rushing blood in the access). If you don't "feel the thrill," or it feels extremely low, please get a stethoscope and call the nurse or another technician to double-check your findings. Some patients have accesses that work, but the thrill is extremely low, meaning the connection of blood flow for dialysis is really deep below the skin. So make sure, especially if this is your first time cannulating that patient.

You must always be on your game in terms of evaluating the access. Look for redness, previous infiltration swelling, hot-to-touch feel, peeling, blisters, and bleeding. Document this, and inform the nurse of these findings. This evaluation should take one to two minutes, not ten minutes, unless you're having trouble "feeling the thrill" or "hearing the bruit."

Complications

If the access is extremely hot to the touch, or red, it could be infected with...what? I don't know. Only the doctors know. Don't stick the patient, period, without informing the nurse. He/she may be able to call the doctor and get an order for antibiotics, or the doctor may want to send the patient out for access evaluation, or to the hospital. If the patient's arm has been previously infiltrated from the last treatment, talk to the nurse then remember to go above the infiltrated area, not into it, because that would create more swelling. Some clinics say no sticking around the area at all because that area can continue to swell even though you go above that swelling. If swelling is all over the site, then ask if the patient still feels pain and ask the nurse where it would be best to stick if the nurse/doctor gave permission for that patient to still be put on the machine.

The best method for infiltration is rotated hot and cold packs, but follow your unit's protocol regarding this. If the access is clotted, you'll know, because the bruit or thrill will be absent. If you're definitely sure neither of those signs is present, then you really need to use a stethoscope and call a nurse or another technician to double-check your findings. Then the patient's assigned medical doctor should be called, and the patient may be sent to an access intervention center or vascular doctor to fix the access. Many times, after the access receives intervention, the vascular doctor or center will send the patient back to the dialysis clinic to receive treatment the same day, depending on the findings and intervention received.

Step 2 - Cleaning the Access

Every unit is so different in their protocols. Again, whatever they say—do it. Usually, you will take two alcohol pads or a Betadine if your patient is allergic to one or the other. You'll cleanse only the spot you're sticking, not the whole arm. You're trying to minimize the number of bacteria on the surface of the needle sites before you stick the patient, because you don't want to carry those germs with the needle into the bloodstream.

68

Some technicians feel this is the opportunity to clean the whole arm instead of just the two needle sites, and this is a big no-no. It's said in some units that you should stick the patient when the alcohol is wet on the skin instead of dry, but many patients refuse, insisting they don't like it. As for Betadine, some units say two to three minutes to dry on the skin before you stick. If you have patients who refuse clinical methods, document all refusals every time and notify the nurse.

Allergies

Some patients have allergies to the paper tape. If so, look for plastic tape or cloth tape. However, these are really adhesive tapes that can tear the skin when removing them pre- or post-treatment. When removing these extremely adhesive tapes, wet a 2 x 2 gauze pad with alcohol, or get an alcohol pad, and wet the parts of the tape not touching the dressings. If you don't, it can scar the patient or tear the patient's skin off when you take it off posttreatment. Tell the patient to purchase a bottle of alcohol for 99 cents so that if they keep the dressing on after treatment then taking it off won't ruin their skin or make it difficult to get off tape marks. See Figure 3.

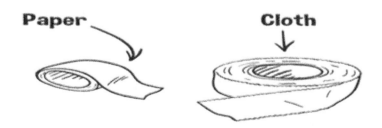

Figure 3

Hairy Arms

Some patients have really hairy arms, and there's a certain way to tape their lines after you cannulate them. You should tape the lines up and away from the hairs on their access. Tape the lines to the upper part of their shirt, or use clamps to redirect their line. Never tape lines on hair because when you take off the tape you'll definitely hear sounds of discomfort, or even shouts of profanity. See Figure 4 below.

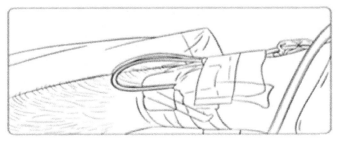

*Figure 2 :*Tape up the lines up away from the hair.

Step 3 - Cannulating

Hmm…This is that part that most patients dread, the "who's sticking me today" part. When you're about to stick the patient, always stretch the skin a little and slowly push the needle in. Using this method, I've been told by many patients that this technique is a winner because they don't really feel any pain at all. I don't jerk or shove the needle in, or push the needle in too fast, or the patient will be in pain and may not want me to stick them next time. Even with my ease in method, some patients say that my method is no good and prefer someone else to stick them, which isn't a problem for me. I'm not perfect, but I always try my best to minimize pain at all times. But, honestly, needles will always hurt when penetrating skin, so just know that. See Figure 5 on the next page.

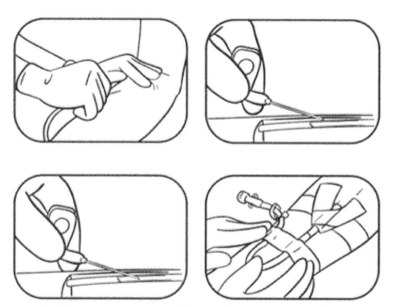

Figure 5: *Remember stretch the skin and slowly insert the needle*

Wait, Don't Stick Me!

Some patients may not want you to be near them, or cannulate them, for various reasons. No matter what, listen to the patient and immediately notify the person they request to cannulate them. Please don't argue with the patient that you are a good cannulator or you have experience. I've seen this happen over and over. Listen—if the patient says, "No, DON'T STICK ME," that's what they mean. I'll repeat this in my chapter on per-diem tips! This is one of the reasons staff members gets cursed out, including me when I was just starting out: NOT LISTENING!

Cursing or any type of verbal abuse coming from the patient shouldn't be tolerated by staff, but this is one reason this abuse happens. It's the patient's body. How are you going to demand what you want to do with their body? If the patient wants me to stick in an area I know is clearly off limits according to clinical protocols, like their access is really huge and shiny and they want me to stick right in the shiny part, I kindly say I can't and explain why. Either I offer another site on the arm that is safe to cannulate, or I call someone else, or the nurse, to stick the patient. And I document this.

Know-It-All Technicians

I repeat! Many technicians want to show off instead of calling another technician who can get the needle in correctly. They'd rather bluff about their years of experience, and force the patients to let them stick them— or they may catch an attitude with that patient. I sometimes have a patient who refuses me for whatever reason and requests that I call over another technician. Guess what? I continue to respect them and I ask if there's anything else they need, and bam, it's a done deal.

Please, listen to the patients, not that they're always right, but neither are we, so it's best to be mutually respectful, especially if they just came out of surgery to receive a new, transformed access or to get the access repaired. The doctor has given them special instructions in order to maintain that access for a long period of time. Listen to the instructions the doctor sent to them to give to you on where you should not to go, and where you are allowed to go, and life will be easier. They will appreciate and thank you many times for your respect.

Experienced Certified Technicians' Tips for Newbies

Dash, Jose, and Debbie (names changed to protect identity) are experienced technicians and have offered advice to newbies.

When you come in as a newbie, you have the privilege to be looked upon as someone who is saving lives, and is in a job to improve patient's lives, not make them miserable. If you're getting into this profession you should understand that you must be sympathetic and understanding. Many patients bring a lot of issues into the clinic because they have stuff going on at home and they're also angry that their kidneys no longer function like yours. You need to understand how they feel and sympathize with them, but at the same time not put up with abuse from them. - **Dash**

I've seen technicians begin doing too much to please others, and I've even reached out to tell them that they shouldn't be doing stuff outside of their job description in the facility (mopping behind the machine, stocking, and other stuff). Those same newbies ignore this important advice. They don't know that the rest of the staff hates it when a person does work outside their job description because they fear that their manager will make those extra duties mandatory. Stop trying to please people and do your job, which is to care for patients, not trying to get the attention of others by trying to impress them when you're only making yourself look like a fool. -**Jose**

I feel that new dialysis technicians should humble themselves and take advice from older, experienced technicians who have been around. Many new technicians

I've seen have come into the unit as know-it-alls instead of learning-it-alls and it is frustrating. I recall an incident where this technician was just starting off and within a year he felt as if he owned the place and was shouting directives and being inappropriate to staff, patients, and to me. **-Debbie**

Past Clinical Managers' Advice

A big issue I noticed in dialysis is that sometimes the staff isn't all that sympathetic with the patients and brings those attitudes from their own homes and dumps them on the patients, and I hate that. These patients don't have kidneys that work—you do—and you should treat them with the utmost respect and always keep that in mind.

- T. Showers

Becoming a patient care technician is a great way to learn the dos and don'ts in dialysis. As a newbie, I encourage you to rotate your section. It makes you a better technician and allows you to develop skills and techniques on the best ways to cannulate different accesses. I would also encourage you to utilize this role as a steppingstone to advancing your career. Be open to opportunities offered to you by the clinical manager. Go to any classes that the facility offers. These classes are opportunities you need to propel you forward. Don't worry initially about whether you are getting paid to be a preceptor, to attend classes, or to go to an outside clinic to view a procedure. All these experiences will benefit you in the long run. Stay away from the gossip and the negative staff. They will only bring you down.
- Dyline

Past Educator Advice

Listen to your patients because you can tell how their day is going and your listening is important to them. Also, limit going away from your patients into another technician section to sit down and chat when you should be monitoring them. I've seen cases where some patients pass out very quickly and it's important to monitor them properly. **-R. Davis**

Things You Should Understand About the Job

1. You don't have to move slowly to know what you're doing. You should move at a good pace with 100% understanding of what you're doing and why.

2. I know the money offered at the interview table sounds good, but if you don't have empathy or passion for this work, refuse the job.

3. You are known by your skills and how you treat people. Dialysis is a small world. You never know who knows whom and whom you may need as a contact in the future.

4. Know your patients. Always ask if they've had any complications since their last treatment, because they may be suffering in silence.

5. Don't argue with or be disrespectful to management, no matter how crazy you think they are, because the day you do can be your last day. And always document!

6. Always go in twos or threes to management to discuss any disagreements with staff or patients, especially if you have no union. You need a witness!

7. Never let any job stress you more than your own family issues stress you.

CHAPTER #7
MY EXPERIENCE WITH EXPERT JOSE

"Excellence is to do a common thing in an uncommon way."
- Booker T. Washington

I recall when I didn't know too much about venturing out into other units. I wanted to learn more and more about dialysis but was stuck and didn't know how to go about it. I remember this very nice Puerto Rican guy coming into the unit. From the time he came in until the time he left, everyone loved and adored this technician, from staff to patients. I didn't understand why my own patients were calling out to him as if they were losing their minds, wanting him to put them on the machine. They would shout, "Jose! Jose! Hey, man, what's up? Are you working over here? I hope you are!" When I told my patients that he was busy and that I would have to put them on, they were vexed like never before. I was confused and kind of baffled. (I soon understood that some of my patients considered me slow and just an average technician when I asked them about my skills.) I didn't understand what was going on and what was so special about Jose. I began observing him to figure out what he was doing differently from what I was doing. I noticed he was fast and did things properly, and he was very cool with all his teammates. I never saw him have an issue with anyone. At this point, I wasn't jealous, just curious. After all, he was friendly and extremely helpful, so I sucked up enough courage to ask him one day about his secrets to receiving so much positive attention.

This guy spilled the delicious beans about his celebrity dialysis attention. Because of this, I have never again been an average technician. He came from another unit that was tougher. Things were out of order there, so he had to be intelligent, superfast, and knowledgeable. He overcame a whole lot on his own in the past as a newbie under an expert technician who allowed Jose to shadow him. Jose told me how that preceptor was the bomb, how he just observed whatever he did and asked questions at the end, and how much genius stuff he learned. The stuff he told me blew my mind because it was common sense that should've been implemented from the get-go. Hey, I didn't know. But I do now.

Because of Jose, I was able to work in other units with the same rock star results, invited back time and time again to work per diem. On top of that, patients were very excited to see me and asked me to be put them on the machine. In the chapter titled "Perdiem," I'll share different comments I received because of following Jose's Way. I've listed a few of his powerful secrets on the next page.

8 Powerful Secrets I Learned From Jose

1. **Humbleness is KEY!** Be friendly with the patient at all times. Many times you can turn rude, noncompliant patients into those who ask you to put them on the machine. You'll build exploding trust if you put your attitudes aside when they give you theirs.

2. **Put patients FIRST and computers LAST**. This was the part that really had many patients requesting me to tend to them. I stopped wasting time the minute Jose told me this. I asked the patient, once seated several important questions, took their vitals, evaluated their access, THEN cannulated the patient and started treatment on the machine. After that, I found a teammate to provide a second signature and other information to start treatment on the electronic paper. Jose showed me how I should always deal with the patient first before playing around with the electronic paper.

3. **Teamwork.** This is a very important lesson he shared. He told me that he worked as a team with a few motivated dialysis technicians, that they were the bomb, and that not all of them wanted to be a team. Instead, they wanted to hate on him and cause problems because every patient loved Jose, and a couple of technicians became jealous. So, Jose taught me how to teamwork swap. If a patient refuses me, I go to him or a teammate and explain it, then I suit up to take care of his patient while he or another tech deals with mine. He also taught me the double-up, as I call it. When your teammate needs help, both of you work on one or the other's patient at the same time to put them on. One technician works on the machine information while the other cannulates the patient. They go from patient to patient together, the patient gets on in three minutes, and treatment begins. Hmm...Wow, I was so excited.

4. **Help your teammates.** In other matters besides direct patient care, I noticed Jose would sometimes clean all

the patient chairs of another technician. I didn't want him to do it, but he told me the reason why. He did that favor because if he became worn out and couldn't clean his chairs that technician would render him the same favor because they had worked it out between them. Jose would also set up a machine or put on a patient for other teammates but only for those who rendered the same favors to him. He also showed me how not to be a dummy and do all the work for someone who is too lazy to help you the same way in return. Whatever he did, it was balanced.

5. **Shut up and listen to management**. I noticed that most of my issues in the past stemmed from anger with management issues. No matter how crazy the different managers acted, or what they said, or how they acted, Jose always retained his composure. He was quiet during staff meetings and always said yes when they asked, "Do you all understand?" He said that getting angry and losing your source of bread and butter isn't worth it and he preferred it that way, stress free. A manager even told me in the past to follow Jose's Way of being quiet in the meetings; because that's the reason she felt he was the best.

6. **Be a CLEAN technician**. Don't do the patch method, like taping gauze on an arm that's bleeding while the patient is on the machine. Remove the bloody tape and put on fresh tape, and always put alcohol in your post packs so you can clean the patient's arm. Don't let them leave dirty or messy. You want to return their arm in better condition than they gave it to you.

7. **Have passion for your work**. Jose showed me he's passionate in working with his patients. It's very important to him, and the way others portray him to the patient matters deeply to him. One time Jose was misrepresented by staff in front of a patient and I witnessed him turn very red and become upset because of it. He went into the restroom, calmed down, and regained his composure. He came back in a calm mood and straightened out that mess, all while being professional with the patient.

8. **Don't do everything for everybody**. Jose explained that certain duties outside my job description shouldn't be done. I shouldn't become overworked and tired by doing work outside the scope of my job, especially for people who won't help me in return.

"HELP I am alone on the floor"! 7 Quick Tips

If you just came on the floor after all of the patients are on, and you are certified and trained but nervous about what to do, here are some tips.

1. Find out what section you will be in.

2. Introduce yourself to each of your assigned patients and ask if there is anything they may need.

3. Monitor your patients or ask for assistance in doing so.

4. Look at your patient's machines and get the times they will be coming off.

5. Educate yourself in advance on where everything is located in the center.

6. Stack your section with pre/post supplies and packs. I will talk more about how to make them in the next chapter.

7. I repeat again, humble yourself and listen to the patient because this is where you gain a lot of expert knowledge.

CHAPTER #8
QUICK PRE- & POSTTREATMENT PROTOCOLS

You have a choice: You can either hate on motivated people or learn from them.

This is a very important chapter because the methods explained are timesavers; however, don't follow any protocols without making sure your company or clinic uses these practices. I stress and stress this because I know people are quick to sue for simple reasons and statements, and I'm simply expressing here what I've seen and experienced. So please be aware that this is not listing any company's confidential protocols or procedures. This is just a simple style shown to help patients.

Now that you've gotten a taste of what dialysis is like in terms of patient access evaluation and complications, and tips from others and me in the dialysis field, I'll give you a spoonful of how to make ten to thirteen hours of your day extremely productive and less stressful. I've worked per diem in over six units. I have to say again and again, organization is extremely crucial, because when faced with turnover you absolutely must know how to properly and professionally discontinue old shifts and put on new patients for the new shifts. You must know how to safely pull-out needles without blood spilling everywhere, and you must make sure your next-in-line shift patient gets on the machine at a reasonable or scheduled time.

Remember, how you put on your first shift patients affects the next shift of patients and can basically hurt or help your day. If you put on all early morning patients late then everyone the rest of the day will be late. Same fact goes for patients who get on in good time.

Some units have scheduled times and designated chairs for patients but, honestly, I've had no success in the implementation of scheduled times—because stuff happens. If your patients are coming in late, find out why. Maybe their transportation should be changed, or other factors can be the reason for lateness. First of all, every unit, whether private or corporate, is completely different. Take the time to learn their different protocols and procedures early on, especially if you're working there per diem. Some units, not all, will allow you to pull out the patients who have finished treatment and are still holding their access to fill that spot with a new shift patient so the rest of the shift won't be affected.

Hand Washing/PPE Alert

You won't believe that I've seen staff that don't gel or wash their hands until they're going on break. This is disgusting and dangerous. Several times in the past I've witnessed staff who put on a pair of gloves, discarded the posttreatment lines on the machine, cleaned the machine, and put a new setup there, all while wearing the same old dirty gloves. Please, don't ever do that! By the way, those folks were fired! Wash/gel your hands all the time, especially before, in between, and after treating the patient.

MRSA (Methicillin-resistant Staphylococcus aureus) is transmitted by healthcare workers who don't wash their hands, and I've witnessed this problem again and again in different units. Some coworkers will even save the gown or apron they've used that day to wear for the next couple of weeks or months. That's really nasty. Every day we pick up new germs and those gowns should be thrown away. If you have a plastic shield and blood gets on it, you can wash it off with bleach, but anything like cloth gowns should be thrown away before going home, not saved for the next day or any day.

Starting Your Day, Especially if You're Late

Let me emphasize how to start your day: Follow the "Quick Treatment Protocol" and make "winner" packs. Before coming to the unit I usually pray for a smooth day, without any issues in the clinic or on the floor, but I've listed on the next page what you should do.

First Things First

1. Locate a clean gown, gloves, and shield.

2. Go your section.

3. Prepare chairs first (putting a sheet on the chair if none is spread out). The reason I emphasize this is because if you're running late and patients are coming in, you need sheets spread first so patients can sit down and wait for you to tend to them. Make a hole in the near top of a sheet and hook it to the near top handle on the back of the chair instead of wasting time tying it. Plus, using this

method makes the sheet stay secure in the chair instead of sliding off.

4. Be sure your machine is primed and any tests, including phoenix meters, are completed.

5. If you have packs made, put them on the chair or side tables connected to the chair, if allowed.

6. You should wear/change gloves when touching the machine and dealing with the patient in between—which I will be discussing below. Again, hand washing is super important.

If you have a patient who doesn't want or require assistance weighing on the floor scale and comes in directly to their chair, ask, "How are you doing, Mr./Mrs./Ms. X? Any complications?" However, some unit's say all patients should be weighed by a staff member to be sure the weight is correct so you don't remove too much and the patient cramps in pain on the machine.

Now, WHILE you are putting on the blood pressure cuff, put in the treatment information on the machine (time running, fluid goal, and volume). I emphasize, don't waste valuable time fooling around with other stuff. Please take the blood pressure first, find out the weight (if you didn't weigh the patient), ask if they had any complications last time, and put this in the electronic computer, all while the blood pressure is being taken. Then evaluate the access and stick the patient. Many technicians fail here; Jose taught me that! You shouldn't be fooling around with the computer or paper after the blood pressure has been taken and the patient is waiting! You should put only weight, normal blood pressure, and temperature in the computer, and then go back to it after the patient is on. These people have lives and are waiting to complete their treatment in their prescribed time.

Repeat, because it's IMPORTANT!!

Don't drag around and wait for the electronic paper before starting treatment, because coworkers sometimes run late to work and other teammates can be very busy putting their patients on and can't give you a double (a second signature).So just put three to four pieces of information (weight, temperature, blood pressure, and respiration) into the electronic sheet or paper sheet, then come back after your patient is on, then start treatment on the ELECTRONIC PAPER. If you don't use electronic paper, only regular pen and paper, that's even better. This is different from starting treatment on the machine. You should press Start Treatment on the machine immediately after hooking up the patient to the machine. Once the blood that was cleaned from the machine flows back into the patient's body that's when treatment usually begins. But always check with your clinic first to be sure you're doing the right thing.

Weight & Goal

Each kilogram is equal to 2.2 pounds. Know this: When a patient tells you, please don't remove 3 kg (which is 6.6 lbs.) because of cramping during previous treatments at that goal amount, please listen and understand them. Don't say, "Well, you're over your dry weight and I'll have to set the machine to take off 4.4 kg. I've seen cases where the patient became very ill on the machine because of this and the technician had to discontinue treatment. I find that most companies have a protocol where they tell staff they must put in whatever goal the computer says without verifying it with the patient before each treatment.

This, to me, is horrible. This tells me I'm setting the goal against the patient's wishes, making it harder for them to sustain the treatment because of cramps. And guess what? The worst part is that the patient skips treatment the next time to avoid discomfort again. Many times, the dry weight goal in the chart should be adjusted, but isn't. Always verify with the patient how much you're taking off. Say, "I'm taking off X number of kilograms, which is equal to Y pounds. Are you okay with this?" It really makes the patient feel at ease and able to trust you. The doctor is the one who adjusts the fluid goals of the patient, but sometimes doctors are unreachable. You must use your judgment cautiously, and consult with the nurse.

Patients Calling

Sometimes patients call me out of my section to complain or to tend to them because their technician has taken too long to put them on. I used to take forever because I accepted advice from everyone; as a result, everyone's words were swimming in my head. Well, this continual calling for me made me frustrated about why other technicians didn't accept the idea of "patient first," but did accept "to each his own." This is a bother sometimes because I get so busy with my own patients, but I still cater to those patients who personally request me.

Some technicians get jealous and don't understand why patients continue to call and call me when they are present or at the patient's side. It's Jose's Way of "patient first and computer after." At times, I have run late. I remember getting to work ten minutes late, but do you know, I put on all my patients within thirty minutes as if I hadn't been late. Other technicians were putting on their first or second patient at the time I was finished and starting treatment on the electronic sheet.

Next, I will review Quick Treatment Protocols.

Quick Treatment Pre protocol

- Greet patient.

- Put on blood pressure cuff while going over weight, complications, and taking their temperature, all at the same time.

- Put only those three to four things into the computer or electronic paper until you are finished with the patient.

- Evaluate the access and cannulate the patient.

- After patient(s) is started on the dialysis machine then quickly finish writing, electric charting, and/or computer work.

Refer to chart, Figure 6 below

Advantages and Disadvantages of the Quick Treatment Pre
protocol

ADVANTAGES	DISADVANTAGES
Patients will love and appreciate this	Some staff won't understand your new technique
Makes Life easier for you	Patients will call you all the time, because their technician isn't using this protocol
You have rare knowledge	Some patients will be a bit upset that your aren't their tech
Your 2nd 3rd and 4th shifts will get on and off on time depending if they come in on time	Can be overwhelming when most patients are calling you

Figure 6

Quick Treatment Protocol Information

Patients will love and adore you for this! You'll be the best to them and they'll always want you because you care for them first. Here's my advice for Quick Treatment Protocol for posttreatment. It's good to time yourself for seven minutes, and seven minutes only, starting after the patient has been rinsed back, to the time you take out the needles. Afterward, the patient may have blankets to fold and perhaps other necessities that are out of your hands (talking to neighbor patients while hogging the chair). Understand that the post protocol is putting information first and the patient second, because occasionally electronic sheets freeze and information from the machine sometimes can't be recovered if you wait too long. The patient is still first in this method, but in a creative way. So, it's wise to be sure you get all the information out of their machine, and I mean everything. If they're a real bleeder then you have to be patient and give them a glove so they can hold their access, or you hold it because a great loss of blood can make them very anemic.

Don't rush anything but know your stuff. Okay, time is approaching for that patient's treatment to come to an end. They have about five minutes left, so let's determine how you're going to utilize those crucial minutes. First of all, you should have taken the ending times of all your patients on your downtime. With that information you should have a good idea of how to properly flow for that shift. Example: Patient Z is coming off in three minutes but you also have Patient A coming off in twenty minutes, and so on and so on. You would know if you can squeeze in another patient on the second shift behind Z if you can get her out of the chair before A comes off. If you know that Z has a few minutes left, you should definitely open the electronic chart or use your paper and prepare to take the post temperature, respiration, sitting blood pressure, and patient well-being. Put that in the chart after the "finish" alarm rings.

It should be less than two minutes by then. That will give you time to take any additional blood pressure for your ending treatment, and determine if the pressure is stable. Now the machine alarm has rung for Z to come off. Your next move should be to initiate whatever blood pump flow speed your protocols tells you to rinse back the patient, and you should be putting in all the post information, such as ending blood flow rate and other results from the machine, or putting the blood work into the paper or electronic chart.

In instances when the patient isn't feeling well, you should do all you can for the patient and notify the nurse, but clean the machine and set up a new set ASAP! You should let that patient recover. If the BP still won't improve, tell the nurse and ask if it's okay to give salty broth (to raise BP) or move the patient to the side, within your view, to be sure she/he recovers, depending on whether you have unit permission or not. If you're a newbie starting off, just give yourself time to learn what to do and don't rush anything if you are unfamiliar with what you're doing.

Initiating the Quick Treatment Postprotocol

Now back to Patient Z's needles. I'll share several methods with you.

Method #1

You'll need 1 packaged sterile 4x4 and 2x2 gauze, with two pieces inside; 1 alcohol set; 1 small roll of tape; bandage; your size gloves; and 2 large blue chucks. First, put one chuck under the patient's access arm, then tear off six strips of tape and stick them on the side of the table chair, or pull it directly from the roll. Some units allow you to use the 2x2 sterile gauze before you place a bandage on the site; if so, fold your sterile 2x2 gauze the TINIEST you can and pull out the needle a little and place the gauze close to the insert spot where the needle remains. Many technicians don't fold it as tiny as possible and the patient bleeds through. Put your two bandages on top as you hold the folded 2x2 gauze in place, then take your 4x4 gauze and fold it really tight and as small as you can to create a great holding bond, then pull the needle into safety snap, if you have one, and press down.

Put around 3 to 4 strips of tape on each holding bond spot, and if the patient requests it, you should remove the tape after less than ten minutes of holding. When you press down, don't press down to stop the flow of blood in and out of the access. Hold the gauze in a semi hard position. If you press/tape the gauze down too hard and long, you can stop the blood from flowing through the access and clot it, and that's definitely not good. Some patients want both needles out at the same time, and that's really up to you and the unit's discretion. Sometimes, if you aren't careful when you take out two at the same time, one of the sites can start bleeding because of the pressure you're putting on the other needle site.

Method #2

You'll need 1 package sterile gauze with two pieces inside; 1 alcohol set; 4 bandages or 2 sure-seal; your size gloves; one large glove for the patient; and 2 large blue chucks. You will pull the patient's needle into the safety cap and press down on the site with one tightly rolled 4x4 gauze so it won't bleed. Give the patient the large glove so they can hold the access. When they stop bleeding, put the bandages on top of the site and nothing else.

Using the first method of folding the gauze and putting it on the needle sites was one of the best methods allowed at many clinics. The patients love it and are ready to get out of the chair in ten minutes or less because the 2x2 gauze serves as a great barrier under the bandage to stop the bleeding. After both methods, alcohol should be used to clean the patient's arm of any blood residue. Many patients I encounter love the first method. They say the bleeding time is less for them.

Refer to chart, Figure 7.

93

ADVANTAGES	DISADVANTAGES
In most cases, less bleeding	Some clinics don't allow this technique
Patients will get out of the treatment chair faster	Some patients refuse this
Many patients prefer this	Doesn't always work for everyone

Figure 7

Nursing Home Patients

I suggest that you never bandage a nursing home or wheelchair-bound patient and send them out the door without first making sure that they have stopped bleeding, and change the bloody bandages—don't leave them on. I've seen this happen; however, I found out that when you tape up those patients without checking and cleaning the post mess off the patient's arm, like bloody bandages, it's dangerous. Example: Ms. B, an elderly nursing home patient, comes in and out on a stretcher. This particular day she has finished her treatment of four hours a bit early, cutting her treatment by twenty minutes. Since she has gotten off the machine early, it messes up that technician's flow for that shift. Ms. B is now coming off at the same time as two other patients on that row, which is three and a half hours long, and it will be difficult to get everyone off at the same time.

Pressed for time, this technician doesn't hold her needle sites but tapes her access super tight and sends her on her way without checking to see if she's still bleeding, or replacing the bandages with fresh gauze and tape. On the way back from dialysis, the patient begins to bleed through the tight bandages. The EMT transport sees this; Ms. B loses a lot of blood on the way back to the nursing home. Now she must go on to the hospital where she will be hospitalized because of the huge blood loss, plus she now needs a transfusion.

Another scenario can be that the nursing home staff doesn't follow through and remove the old bandages from the access. This allows bacteria to grow on the access and seep into the needle site hole that is healing. Some patients come back to dialysis with blisters or slightly red skin from the bandages staying on since the last treatment. Please clean those sites really well if you ever encounter that kind of case—and document it.

I want to reflect again on what is required to make winner "put on" and "take off" packs. These packs are important and should be made up on your downtime after all patients are started on their machines. I'm simply explaining this method; create your own style.

Here's what you'll need to make pre- and post-packs. Remember; follow your clinical protocols in everything.

See Figure 8 for a picture of a pre- and post-pack.

Method Reflection

PRE

Your needle set: 14-, 15-, 16-, or 17-gauge needles

2 Alcohol pads or 2 Betadine

Your gloves inside 2 "chucks" or blue pads

1 roll of tape

POST

1 alcohol set of 2 pads (to wipe and clean the patient's arm)

1 4x4 set of two gauze

1 2x2 small gauze (depending on your unit)

1 to 2 small rolls of tape

2 "chuck" or blue pads. Your gloves inside

Wrap up your packs with a piece of tape and put them by your section or in the cabinet.

Remember: When you're about to cannulate the patient, always put one chuck under the patient's arm and work off the second chuck, meaning put all pre- or post-supplies on one chuck while you are preparing the patient for cannulation. When finished, remove the second chuck with the leftover materials just used, and put it in the trash. The chuck under the patient's arm shouldn't be soiled with blood, but if it is please replace it with a clean one. If the chuck isn't soiled, leave it there until posttreatment. The post pack you bring should include a chuck you can work off of and discard once you're finished. Never leave trash with the patient.

Educate

Explain to all your patients with fistula or graft accesses the importance of taking care of their lifeline. If the patient leaves the bandages on until the next treatment, bacteria can grow under the bandage. It can cause infections, clotting, and other problems for the access. Find out your unit's policies regarding educating the patients on properly caring for their access before and after treatments.

Packs

Limit running back and forth to retrieve supplies from the counter and cabinets unless your unit has a supply/drawers protocol. Make up your packs, prepare your bleach cloths, and make lines and dialyzers accessible. Not doing so is a crucial time waster. You can put an individual ready-made pack by the patient or on top of the machine ONLY if your clinic allows you to do so. If not, just put them all in a box or container and store it close by. I find it shocking that some coworkers don't do anything on their downtime then struggle over and over during turnover. This is ridiculous and can cost your second, third, and even fourth shifts to get on the machine late, making you go home more stressed, tired, and unhappy. You want to clock out tired—but not overworked.

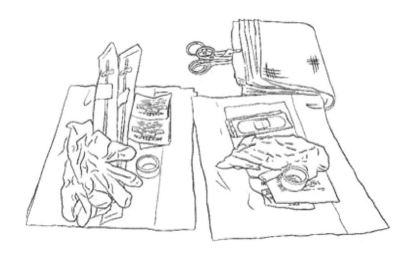

Figure 8

Now reflect on those methods above and try your best to implement them if your clinic allows. If the clinic doesn't allow you to set packs on the counter, put them in a box to get them off the counter. Or, if the clinic won't allow you to prepare packs ahead, ask them what to do so you will be on your A+ game.

Wasting Supplies Is a NO-NO

A few teammates could do better in terms of conserving supplies. I've notice unnecessary supplies that aren't being used, being placed inside of pre and post packs. I've seen eight or more individual pieces of gauze in their post pack, or 3-4 whole rolls of tape, and excessive blue chucks. Please, don't be a waster. Be smart and find out by observing your patient what is needed and what is not. Some patients bleed a lot and some don't, so for the bleeders you'll put a little more gauze in your pack to prepare for any heavy bleeding. But don't put so many supplies in your pack for patients who don't bleed a lot.

CHAPTER #9
CRITICAL SITUATION
QUESTIONNAIRE

*You've got to be kidding. Telling a lie doesn't cover you
—only the truth of a situation will.*

I've heard and seen some extremely crazy situations. In tough times, I still do what is right, but in the past, I initially took the wrong advice. I didn't break any policies but saw things that I should've spoken up about. Now that I'm older and wiser, no one can pull the wool over my eyes concerning the right thing to do. I want you to reflect on certain nonfiction situations and decide what you would do in each instance.

Situation #1 - A disgruntled technician sticks an unruly patient the wrong way and blows up the access, making the needle site and arm so infiltrated that he can't continue treatment. When the tech realizes what's happened, the tech asks you for help.

Would you:

A. Tell the manager

B. Tell the nurse and then tell the manger

C. Keep it to yourself

D. Talk to the technician

E. Different answer/none of the above

Situation #2 - You witness a technician very tightly tape up a severely bleeding patient. The technician doesn't clean up the patient, but simply piles more bandages on top of the bleeding mess. After the bleeding appears to stop, the technician doesn't clean the arm or replace the bandages but says, "Okay, you're good to go!" Would you:

A. Tell the manager

B. Tell the nurse and then tell the manger

C. Keep it to yourself

D. Talk to the technician

E. Different answer/none of the above

Situation #3 - A patient eats heavy food while on the machine and chokes; the food is lodged in his throat. Would you:
A. Perform the Heimlich maneuver.

B. Tell the nurse and then tell the manger.

C. Recline patient and open the saline bag.

D. Perform the Heimlich maneuver & call the nurse and nearby technicians.

E. Different answer/none of the above.

Situation #4 - A technician calls you over to help stick the patient in another spot, takes the needle out of the arterial, and sticks the same dirty needle into another area. Would you:

A. Document this.

B. Tell the nurse and then tell the manger.

C. Keep it to yourself.

D. Talk to the technician.

E. Different answer/none of the above.

Situation #5 - A patient with a mental disability pulls out his access needles; blood is everywhere and it's a mess. Would you:
A. Stop the machine.

B. Tell the nurse and then tell the manger.

C. Stop the machine and clamp all dialysis lines.

D. Keep it to yourself.

E. Different answer/none of the above.

Situation #6 - A nurse working as a technician fills in the patient's entire posttreatment information (blood volume processed, blood flow rate, dialysis flow rate, blood pressure, temperature, and weight) before the patient ends the treatment. When the patient weighs, the nurse says, "Okay, 'bye!" Would you:
A. Tell the manager.

B. Talk to the nurse and then tell the manger.

C. Keep it to yourself.

D. Tell another technician.

E. Different answer/none of the above.

Situation # 1

Answer D. Talk to the technician

It's best to communicate with your teammate in asking what is really going on. Even if they may give you attitude still do it, that way the person knows that you know what's up.

Situation # 2

Answer E. Different answer/none of the above

I see this time and time again, it maybe that technician's technique. I just suggest offering my help to the patient once I witness this.

Situation # 3

Answer D. Call the nurse and nearby technicians, rinse the patient back immediately/have others get crash cart

Situation # 4

Answer D. Talk to the technician

Nine times out of ten that technician knew what they were doing was wrong, and by speaking to that person about how you feel about it is better. It will not be snitching if you did report it or make note of it because you care about the patient, however speaking to people first is my golden rule.

Situation # 5

Answer C. Stop the machine and clamp all dialysis lines

Situation # 6

Answer B. Talk to the nurse and then tell the manger.

You should not feel afraid to speak up about the wrong that you see. That is fraudulent information! This is totally different from a patient forgetting to give you their weight before they leave out of treatment, and you having to calculate it the manual way.

10 Signs of a Good Technician

1. Does their job and follows clinical protocols to the best of their ability. Not unscrupulous.

2. Helps others and is a team player.

3. Goes to classes that help them further their goal of becoming an expert in patient care.

4. Prepares for the next shift on their downtime.

5. Limits gossip and speaking evil of others.

6. Is respectful toward patients and has loads of empathy mixed in with professionalism.

7. Is humble and requests help when needed and is willing to call over another technician when having cannulation issues.

8. Starts treatment for patients in less than ten minutes.

9. Is respectable toward management or apologizes when in error.

10. Seeks to resolve issues in the unit and is part of the solution, not the problem.

CHAPTER #10
DEATH—CAN YOU HANDLE IT?

No one is immune from this word called "death," not even nature.

As I am writing this, I understand that death can hit any of us, in any way possible, at any time. We humans aren't immune to death. However, in the dialysis world, this is a common occurrence because this is the end stage of renal failure. In the beginning of my career as a dialysis technician I was hit very hard emotionally when I heard about the deaths of my dear patients. Upon learning the news, I'd go into the bathroom and bawl because I loved them. Patients that I care for aren't just "anyone" to me; they are awesome patients to me. One patient told a staff member, "Ah, Cassia is too attached emotionally to the patients. That's why she took my best friend's death hard." I have to say I was shocked when I heard such news, and I couldn't help falling apart at home or in the work restroom when I heard of a patient's passing. Now don't think I am saying that all patients with end stage renal failure passes away. I've seen so many patients either get a transplant, or get off of dialysis or improve so greatly while on treatment. So it is possible to have a great life while on dialysis, if the patient continues to adhere to helpful advice from team members, on how to take care of themselves while on dialysis, their life can improve greatly and be sustained.

I recall an incident where a patient told me he was going to pass away that week, and explained how he'd picked out his suit and shaved his head so he would look good in his casket. I told him again and again to stop talking like that, to look for the positive, or talk to the social worker. He refused that, looked into my eyes, and told me he wanted me to come to his wake and funeral. I stood there speechless in disbelief, stunned by his statement. Sure enough, later that week he passed away. On the day of his funeral, after work, I checked myself into SUNY Downstate Hospital, depressed that this came true, that he'd wanted me to attend his funeral, and I couldn't because I had to work. The doctor there gave me the best words ever in terms of encouragement and released me.

Now that I can handle the death of a patient better, I can share this advice: Please prepare yourself to not fall apart emotionally when you hear such news. It hurts, I'm not going to lie about that, and it's okay to cry, and I still do because I really love my patients. I've seen many patients come and go for different reasons. Some had dreams to write a book, go on vacation, do more for their families, or even just to see me the next time—and it never happened.

When their goals disappeared, I was crushed. It's devastating news, but don't let it defeat you. It hurts when you work with someone three times a week and talk with him or her about goals, families, and lives, and suddenly they vanish. That's why I take this job extremely seriously and treat each patient the way, I'd want to be treated. You never know when you're going to say goodbye, or you may not even have that chance.

Brace yourself, as I did and continue to do to this day. Also, in some units, corporate and private, telling patients of the death of another patient is forbidden. To come out and say, "Patient Y died, everybody," is horrible. Some patients' blood pressures shoot up. Some patients pass out upon hearing this news, or have other shock reactions, like intense crying and shaking. Why? Because many of these patients are close friends or have family members on dialysis in the same unit. Many brothers and sisters, cousins, aunts and uncles, even parents, have dialysis in the same clinic and you may never know they're related. Talk about a shock factor.

Sometimes I can handle attending a funeral and sometimes times I can't. It's up to you whether you want to attend a funeral or wake. Learn your clinic's protocol in terms of mentioning death to patients who inquire about other patients. Be strong and strengthen yourself. Don't always be the bearer of bad news, especially in the mornings. If the day is just starting fresh, someone has passed, and you know and want to tell a coworker, wait until the day is almost done. Sometimes a patient may know before staff does for many reasons. Maybe the patient is a relative or rides with that person. If they mention it to you, just express deep condolences in a professional manner, and if you need to step off the floor because of it, again, notify the nurse or a teammate.

7 Ways to Handle Death

1. Tell your coworkers or patients not to mention a death at the beginning of the day.

2. Take deep breaths; calm down.

3. If you're extremely emotional, notify a teammate and go off the floor.

4. Read, listen, or watch something encouraging and uplifting.

5. Take it to a trusted family member or friend.

6. Don't mention a death to other patients until you learn how to do it professionally.

7. If you are strong upon hearing of the passing of a patient but see another teammate is struggling upon hearing the news, comfort them.

CHAPTER #11
MY UNPROFESSIONAL MISTAKES

Some people have diarrhea of the mouth and you just have to hand them the tissue of a closed mouth going forward.

This cautionary chapter tells my mistakes and I wrote it to help you avoid them and be as professional as possible. I didn't have the proper guidance and wisdom that I do now, and although I learned from it, I wish I had known better. I wish I'd had a guide like this when I was starting. Whew! It would have been great.

Old Days

I was very unprofessional, and didn't have the best attitude at times. The following situations showed me that I could change if I allowed it to happen. When I was a dialysis assistant, I flirted and played too much with my patients. Although I didn't think at the time, I would be a dialysis technician in the future, these bad habits came back and bit me in the butt. Years ago, I had one particular patient whose chair I sat near from the time he started treatment to the time treatment ended. We talked about life and joked about a lot of crazy stuff—then he asked me out. I said no because I wasn't interested, and he was offended. He asked, "Is it because I'm on dialysis?" I said, "No, it's not because of that." But I had been too unprofessional and he became very withdrawn and didn't want me to cannulate him once I became a dialysis technician.

In fact, all the patients I had been juvenile with didn't want me to stick them once I became a technician. One said to another technician that she didn't believe I had developed good self-confidence and other issues. It's the worst thing when gossip is spread about you, especially when you're out of line and no one steps up to kindly—I said kindly—tell you what's up. I encourage new, young, or experienced technicians and other staff members to maintain a professional boundary, no matter what. It does matter. When I go into the hospital and a particular nurse or doctor is flirty with me, I don't feel I'll receive the best treatment from them because I don't know what their motives are and I don't feel comfortable discussing my issues.

Lessons Learned

I learned in late 2012 to early 2013 to seriously forgive and move on. A lot of staff issues arise from not forgiving, and I realized I'm getting too old for nonsense. Although words spoken can and are crazy if repeated out of context, gossip is never acceptable in a professional setting. I cried and became angry many times in the staff bathroom when I heard gossip. I've been described as ignorant, crazy, naive southern, and one who has nothing to show for her hard work. All these things shaped me to forgive later on and become a winner over my haters. My advice is to totally avoid gossip. Please, it's not worth it. If you can't say the same sentence to a person's face, don't say it behind his or her back. I used to gossip and the word would come out that Cassia said this and that and the grapevine of lies just kept getting bigger and bigger. Remember, the folks you gossip with and think you can trust will, nine times out of ten, tell your business to someone you wouldn't trust.

No matter how much you try to not acknowledge this about someone you gossiped to, it's true. It's hard, but you can do it. I decided that I wanted to become a better person and speaking negatively about others is not wise, period. It's up to you how you spend your breaks and downtime, and these are merely suggestions based on my experiences.

Doing Too Much For Attention

When I was a newbie, I admit I worked extra hard for everybody to prove myself worthy in their eyes. And guess what? It wasn't worth it. Every time someone's patient was coming off, I'd rush over and do his or her job, cleaning up several other technicians' messes. I see now that I was totally out of control in that area of my work life. A few older technicians told me not to do it but I didn't listen. I was almost worked to death and left every day with more stress than ever. Jose discourages this activity too, because it puts an unfair burden on the technician. Please don't waste your time trying to be popular. Do your job correctly—that's all that matters. I still perform minimum tasks to make sure things stay afloat, such as if I see water on the floor and a housekeeper isn't there, I'll mop it up for safety reasons. If no one brought the supplies for that day, I'll bring them for all my teammates, or at least the teammates in my row. So, I encourage you to pitch in but not to the point where you're taking over someone's job when that person is right there.

Pushed Around

While it's true I was inexperienced, I had and still have the wits to learn and understand how to improve my cannulations, patient care, and professional techniques in general. I hate the bully syndrome and refuse to be bullied by another staff member. Don't let anyone, young or old, licensed or unlicensed, push you into a corner. You can do just as good a job, or even better. Believe in yourself, even if others don't. Show them you're professional by your listening skills, ability to take directions, quick and safe techniques, caring attitude, and your accomplished goals.

I love my older and younger coworkers, but anyone can make a mistake at any time. I've worked with some excellent older technicians who were full of great wisdom and did an awesome job, as well as newbie staff who didn't have much experience but could cannulate and start machine treatment in under ten minutes—plus were good team workers with the desire to continually improve.

Negativity

People withdraw from negative people and you should too, all the while being an awesome team player. The patients are depending on you to create the best treatment experience. Another situation is staff-to-patient issues. One thing I hate is a really bad attitude, especially in the morning. In many units I've been in I've noticed that some people just wake up on the wrong side of the bed all the time. It seldom happens that I'm guilty of this because I claim my day as a good day during meditation in the morning. And it is. I'm not affected by negativity presented by others and you shouldn't either. You've worked hard to get this job and you'd be crazy to let anyone ruin that for you. If you see staff members being extremely rough with patients, you should report them anonymously. If you leave it up to the patient to report it, they sometimes won't for fear of staff backlash and the abuse continues. Several encouraging people at my clinic kept telling me not to give up and to press on. It's vital to let this notion soak in. Don't let anyone make you quit.

My Anger

Once I saw that I was overworking and doing duties outside my workload as a new technician, I quickly became angry. I became even angrier when I heard lies from gossip. I allowed what people say to affect my work and how I treated patients under my care by allowing my hurt to remain secret. I allowed others to make my life a living hell.

Frienemies

As a newbie I confided in the wrong individuals because I couldn't see their hidden hater motives behind the smile. I was too inexperienced to be discerning and didn't know how to differentiate between authentic efforts of help and friendship from other staff members and fake efforts because I was so happy to have a job with good pay. This was one of the biggest mistakes I made. Not everyone is to be trusted. Many people have diarrhea of the mouth where, if you share your situation with them, they keep running to others and telling them such and such said this but "Shh, don't tell anyone else."

Who knows how many people they told not to tell, and those same people turned around and told others. "Shh, don't tell." At times, the people I trusted turned into true enemies, and as a result I didn't say hello because of what I'd heard them say, instead of confronting them about it. Then there were times when I was instructed by my teammates and those in authority to apologize to those I'd confronted unprofessionally, even though I felt I wasn't in the wrong. I took the advice and everything went back to normal in a positive way.

Selling Is a NO-NO

I used to sell Mary Kay and Avon to some patients. Some didn't pay me for whatever reasons and I felt a bit confused and upset. However, I deserved that lesson because I realized later that I was breaking the boundaries of professionalism. The selling had to stop. If a patient didn't pay me, I didn't take it to heart. I continued to treat them well with a nice manner. Everyone isn't good with forgiveness, and if a teammate sells something and never gets his or her money, it can evolve into an unpleasant situation. Please consider this, because I learned too late.

Dating Staff

Personally, I don't like the idea of dating on the job because people somehow know what's up and rumors of sexual relations and other personal aspects begin. I've known staff members who were together before getting their jobs in dialysis. They kept it really professional between them on the job, to the point that you'd never know anything was going on. That was cool. Not everyone has that kind of discipline. If you decide to date or form a relationship with someone on the job, that's your choice; just keep it professional, because if you break up with that person it can create a lot of unhelpful tension in the workplace.

Dating Patients

To me, this is a huge no-no. Many patients have asked me out on dates, and many said, "Shh, no one has to know." You never know if someone will see you together somewhere, the situation then blows up, and you lose your good job. You're there to render professional services to the patients. Some patients I've talked to about this disagree with me; everyone is entitled to an opinion, but this, to me, should not happen. The patients trust you to treat them professionally and you must do so at all times, under all circumstances.

Patients Dating Patients

If patients decide to date other patients, that's really their business, as long as they aren't asking you for personal, private information. Never disclose anything about another patient. That's a serious offense. If the person they're dating finds out that you shared information, he or she can sue your socks off your feet. Beware!

Deep Friendships & Family Ties

I've worked with people in the past that I considered great associates and good friends, but when the lies and gossip circulated, those friendships ended. I've seen this happen to others also, over and over. They may have been friends on the job for a long time then something happens and they're no longer talking anymore. This is not good. Once a friendship collapses, unhealthy tension may enter the workplace. Remember to leave personal business at home, and be professional on the job under all circumstances. Sometimes people are related to others working in the unit. I've heard that families shouldn't be working in the same unit, but it happens. As long as things are professional and no favoritism is in play, I figure all is well.

7 Mistakes Not To Make

1. Skip gossiping about people and being very opinionated.

2. Don't sell small products to the patients.

3. Refuse to fill yourself with negativity.

4. Handle disagreements with other staff and don't allow the job to stress you more than your own situations at home.

5. It's hard but don't hold grudges against patients or staff, try forgiveness. Grudges are so bad for your health and eats up your happiness with revenge.

6. Don't always hang around with other staff members who have unprofessional work habits.

7. Don't speak negative about any co-worker or manager to the patient.

7 Things I'm Proud Of

1. I learned how to develop a professional attitude under all circumstances.

2. I never followed the crowd, even though I was naïve.

3. I learned to choose my battles wisely.

4. I ignored haters and frenemies and realized not everyone always has my best interests at heart.

5. I wrote letters asking for forgiveness to those I wronged and apologized to individuals to keep the peace, even when I wasn't at fault.

6. I understood that if I work toward different goals my family will benefit.

7. I walked away from people who were not good for me, and still maintained professional respect for them.

CHAPTER #12
HECTIC CLINICS

Disorganization can be a career killer once put into daily action.

I've found myself in some really weird situations down through the years while working in many different units. A majority of those units lacked a union. With a union, certain bargaining agreements shouldn't be broken, and staff-to-patient ratio is one of them. In some union facilities, the ratio of patients is three to four per technician and it's against union agreements to have more patients than the technician or nurse should have. In the nonunion units, no strong boundaries exist on how many patients one technician can have; the norm should be three to four patients, but I've seen more and heard that others were constantly under threat of being fired if they were to complain about the situation. A few units are short-staffed, with only four technicians and one nurse for a twenty-four-seat unit. That's where the problems begin.

What if, during turnover, you have someone who passed out on the machine due to not being monitored properly because of lack of staff. How would a technician effectively tend to that patient when he's rinsing back so many people? Or what if a fire occurs and there isn't enough staff to help all the patients escape the blaze? These conditions are truly unsafe and I hope that they're remedied as soon as possible, somehow. In this chapter I'll discuss how to operate in a stressful, hectic center

119

if you decide to work there per diem, or if you're hired there permanently.

I've found some union and nonunion units always remain short-staffed, lack experienced staff, or have a high turnover of staff and management. I've been in a situation where a nonunion unit had twenty patients with only me and another technician and two nurses to treat those patients. So, we split it. I had ten and the other technician had ten, and I put on all my patients in forty minutes. I used a lot of common sense and reasoning to do this. Being in many similar situations helped me gain experience on every level and be a topnotch professional, the best I can be.

In other cases, I recall an electrical shutdown of a dialysis machine while the patient was on and I had to think quickly. What I did at that time worked, and the patient was very pleased that I was his technician when that happened to him. I've had times when all the patients were coming off at the same time and I had all my next shift patients outside waiting for those chairs. I've been in situations where I had only dementia patients and handicapped patients on a shift; that was really tough. I've faced the issue of multiple patients with the same scheduled times assigned to one technician—me. For example, if you have three patients that are three and a half hours long and one patient who is four hours, even if you put them on five or even fifteen minutes apart, it will become very stressful when all their treatments come to an end.

I've listed below several fictional scenarios and described to you how I would handle these critical situations.

Critical situation #1 - You enter a nonunion unit to work for that day and quickly realize that things are disorganized and not all the technicians are there. You see only three technicians, instead of six, and only two nurses. All twenty stations are filled with patients waiting to get on a machine. What do you do in this situation?

First things first: Find out where your section is if you're working per diem. After you've found your section, put on all your assigned patients first before going into any other section. Your assigned section patients must be cared for first, unless the nurse directs you to put on a stick (patient with a graft or fistula) in another section while she/he puts on those one or two catheters you have in your own section. You can then go on to the sections missing a technician, but only if you want to or are instructed to.

First, put the blood pressure cuff on all the patients who aren't on, take their temperature, ask their weight, and whether they had any complications last time. Follow the unit's protocol and, of course, practice hand washing/gel/glove changing in between patients. After you've done that for all the patients you selected to help put on the machines, then go back down the line and follow protocol to start them on the machine and enter the electronic chart/paper chart after they're on.

Critical Situation #2 – Somehow, your patients are backed up to the point where all of them are coming off at the same time—and your third shift is outside waiting for those chairs currently occupied. This unit is short-staffed and the nurse who usually helps you can't because she now has her own assignment of patients. Your patients are upset that their machines are ringing and you're with another patient.

Know who should come off first, second, third, and fourth and go in that order, rinsing them back in the same order. Explain to them while you're taking their information from the machine and rinsing them back that everyone is coming off at the same time and you'll follow the protocol to disconnect them. Emphasize in a calm and professional manner that you haven't forgotten them.

Critical Situation #3 - One of your patients feels very ill when you're rinsing him back, and all your patients are getting off the machine at the same time. Call for assistance from nurses and technicians in a professional manner, and ask for help to rinse back some of your patients because you have an emergency. Also, request a nurse to evaluate that patient.

7 Quick Tips for Hectic Units

1. Don't panic, because the patient will also.

2. Recall all you've learned and put it into action.

3. If the manager is nice and this isn't a union facility, suggest hiring more people. If the answer is no, then limit your per diems there.

4. Evaluate ways to simplify your time there. For example, make packs and double prepare on your downtime.

5. If you work there full time and dislike it, put in applications for other jobs. If you get in somewhere else, then resign, especially if the situation gets really bad in terms of staff-to-patient ratios. Example: 8 patients to 1 technician.

6. Teamwork is precious in critical situations. You and your teammates can double up and put patients on very quickly.

7. On breaks, it really helps offset stress to go outdoors.

5 Things You Never Do in Units

1. Never rinse back multiple patients at the same time.

2. Never add additional time to the treatment time just because everyone will come off at the same time.

3. Never ask another patient to help you with another patient's treatment.

4. Never be rude to the patient because the machine is ringing or their access sites needs assistance.

5. Don't ignore a patient's access trickling blood during and after treatment.

CHAPTER #13
CLINICAL MANAGERS, DOCTORS, & NURSES

A degree in hand lasts a long time, but the way you treat people lasts longer.

Since I've been in dialysis work, I've seen a lot of charge nurses, doctors, and other team members leave the dialysis workforce or transfer out of state. I've noticed there's a high turnover of clinical managers in this profession. After all, the burden of keeping up with sick calls, meeting corporate or private goals each month, and making sure the clinic runs smoothly is exhausting for a clinical manager. Many clinical managers, doctors, and some nurses were joys to work with. I really appreciated them and wished they were still working in dialysis because they were that good in dealing with clinical situations.

Clinical Managers - I've had my share of great and horrible experiences with different clinical managers who filled the shoes of the previous one. I'm listing some quick facts, plus what to look for and how to respect the different individuals over you. Some managers were nice but with a touch of strictness and fairness, and some were flat-out rude, practiced favoritism, and quick to blame you for anything. I've observed some crazy stuff and some horrible situations have happened to me, but believing in myself helped me each time.

My Advice

Clinical managers aren't exempt from the chopping block. I've seen cases where the clinical manager, their supervisor, and the higher supervisor over that one were fired three in a row. If you work with a clinical manager who's treating you unfairly or isn't being compliant with policies and it's affecting you, then call the compliance hotline, document, or take two witnesses with you to confront in a calm way.

3 Reasons for Clinical Manager Turnover

1. Overwork. (Some units don't have administrative assistants and the burden is totally on them.)

2. Stress.

3. Serious company situations.

7 Signs of a Professional Clinical Manager

1. Will tell you the truth about your errors.

2. Can be confided in and is trustworthy.

3. Is organized in terms of the goals and dreams of the unit.

4. Will listen to staff and patients' suggestions, and will institute positive improvements for the clinic.

5. Will help out when the unit is short of staff or a nurse needs a lunch break.

6. Shows staff equal appreciation (suggesting the company sponsor a Christmas lunch, etc.).

7. Doesn't hold grudges or practice favoritism.

5 Signs of an Unprofessional Clinical Manager

1. Doesn't follow up on staff complaints about abusive patients, etc., because they're fearful.

2. Gives preferential treatment.

3. Disregards team-members' personal or family emergencies.

4. Doesn't help out the team.

5. Untrustworthy.

Charge Nurses

My Advice

There are a few great nurses, and then there are some charge nurses and regular nurses who are pushy, disrespectful, and look down on you because you're a technician. If a nurse is treating you unfairly, confront him or her with two witnesses—off the treatment floor—and document, call compliance, or speak to your manager. But, please, be professional about it.

5 Signs of a Helpful Registered Nurse

1. Team player and works with you (taking out needles, helping with patients as needed).

2. On the ball and will initiate patient treatments himself/herself (will put the blood pressure cuff on patients and not wait for you to do it).

3. Knowledgeable and doesn't rely on technicians to tell him/her what to do and how to do it.

4. Professionalism.

5. Organization.

5 Signs of an Unhelpful Registered Nurse

1. Lazy.

2. Unscrupulous.

3. Pressures you to violate unit protocols.

4. Complains to the patients about staff members, management or their personal situations.

5. Practices favoritism.

Doctors

My Advice

I highly suggest you respect them because they have the power to write you up or fire you. If a doctor is unprofessional, talk to the manager about it or call a compliance hotline but, please, document the situation. Some doctors are extremely quiet and only talk to the patient and that's okay. Some are somewhat arrogant and act very unprofessionally. Others are more outspoken and nicer, so please understand this.

5 Signs of a Helpful Doctor

1. Loves and cares for the patients and comes to the unit regularly.

2. Can be reached if the nurse needs an order or a patient needs something.

3. Is respectful of staff and the unit.

4. Listens to technicians regarding the dialysis orders for some patients.

5. Listens to the patients and takes the time to understand how the patients feel about any changes in their orders.

3 Signs You Have an Unhelpful Doctor

1. Patients and staff complain that they can never reach the doctor for a refill of their prescriptions or other issues.

2. The doctor seldom visits his patients to see how they're doing, or to make changes to their dry weight and prescriptions.

3. Ignores staff and doesn't listen to the technician or nurse when they tell the doctor about different issues with the dialysis order that affect the patient.

CHAPTER #14
PER-DIEM TIPS

*Showing your gratitude keeps you in people's heads
longer than just words.*

The mention of the words per diem brings back memories of the energy, youth, and strength I needed to juggle two to three units in one week. I'd be at home location (A) Tuesday, Thursday, and Saturday; location (B) on Mondays; and Location (C) on Wednesday and Friday. Talk about loads of work, but I loved it at the time, especially the huge check at the end of those long two weeks. I worked all over New York City. Extra per diem is where I learned how to be smart, more empathetic, and fast—along with being professional. I've encountered the good, bad, and ugly from working with patients and staff, but all of it shaped me to write this book.

Extensive Experience

Once you're grounded in your unit, I encourage you to venture out and learn the culture of other units while making that mullah cash. This will soften and shape your rough edges and will look great on your résumé. You'll see some units that have technicians who are assigned to only three patients each, or four to five, and you'll see their way of organizing their supplies for turnover, what's allowed there and what's not. You will see technicians who have different techniques and can show you how they make their life easier and, sometimes, what not to do. I've honestly never stopped learning whenever I visit a different unit to do render services. It's because I want to perfect my skills to help others, and you should have that same mindset. No one, and I repeat no one, is perfect, but it never hurts to be smart, quick, neat, and professional. One technician told me that I need to be SLOW in order to be good. I asked him his reasoning, and explained that I can be quick-paced and just as professional, and my results are just as good.

Humbleness

When you go to another center, don't act as if you know everything, even if you're working with someone who doesn't know half of what you know. If you act pushy or like Mr. or Mrs. Know-it-all, you won't get a callback, period. The patients aren't stupid and they know if you're a seasoned technician, new, or pretending to know what you're doing.

Patients will make complaints as well, or straight-out embarrass you by calling loudly for another technician to do the job you can't. To make it easy you should state your name and your clinic to the patient and assure them you know how to put them on the machine properly. Always ask the patients, "May I see your access, and feel it?" When they see that confidence, many times they feel a bit more at ease.

Patients really don't like to see newbies (even if you have years of experience at your clinic, you're still a newbie to them because they've never seen you before at their clinic) for fear that you might infiltrate their access, or maybe they'll experience a lot of pain from someone who's a newbie from another clinic sticking them with needles. If the patient still feels uncomfortable with you after you've felt his or her arm, you calmly ask, "Mrs./Mr. X, would you like me to call someone else to stick your access?" That will make the patient and you feel more at ease with the whole treatment. If you don't ask the patient and attempt to show off, they'll show you off, sometimes screaming or shouting to make you understand that they said, "NO, don't stick me! Do you understand English?!" This is what I've seen and heard in different units.

The patient may shout/scream for another technician or other staff to put them on if you don't follow familiar instructions. It only takes one time for patients to tell me that, and I don't attempt to touch their arm again unless I ask or explain to them that the unit is really short of staff or that their special technician isn't working that day, or is busy.

Also, a patient has told others, "She better not touch me. I don't know where she's from." So, I'm not immune from verbal abuse, but I don't take it personally. I say, "Hi, my name is Cassia from X unit. Who would you like me to call to attend to you, Mr. /Mrs. X?" Many times, because of these manners and the high praise of other patients, that particular patient may just call me over next time and allow me to put them on the machine. Please, listen to the patients. I can't stress this enough. You're working on their arms, not yours, and they many times feel the pain.

Some units that are short-staffed sometimes don't have much choice in hiring a technician to fill in that day. Following is a list of common reasons for not getting a callback from the clinical manager or charge nurse after

133

you've requested overtime at that unit—or a technician may want you to fill in but is prevented from calling you based on the facts below.

16 Reasons You Could Be on the Don't-Call List

1. Really slow—you take more than 10 minutes to put on/take off a patient.

2. Don't listen to patients when they tell you to stop and get someone else.

3. Act like a know-it-all/snappy. (When someone gives you a tip about a patient's likes or dislikes, or cannulation instructions, such as don't go too deep into the access, you ignore them.)

4. Your patients bleed too much posttreatment or complain about you. (You don't clean the patient's arm/garments appropriately if they bleed, or you let them walk out a bloody mess.)

5. Messy technician. (You leave pre/posttreatment supply trash everywhere.)

6. Street like lazy. (You act too cute to attend to patients or do the job appropriately. Not professional.)

7. Breaking rules. (Talking on Bluetooth/playing games on your phone in the unit.)

8. Inappropriate conversations concerning others.

9. Nosing in everyone's business.

10. Taking advantage of the overtime by not clocking out when you have to leave to attend to something and come back.

11. Inappropriate slurs or sexual innuendos.

12. Failure to finish your patient's chart. (Leaving the nurse to sign and finish what you should've done before you left.)

13. Calling out on days the clinic is depending on you to come in.

14. Unit may not want to pay the overtime if you're working within a corporation.

15. Company time stealer. (You were supposed to clock out at your normal time, 7:30 p.m., but stayed until 8:30 p.m., when you were actually finished at 6:50 p.m., to try to get more money)

16. Unit has hired fresh staff and needs no more per diem.

Pay Rate and How to Double Up the Money

Everyone wants to know the pay rates for dialysis technicians because this job compensates well, and if you are in a union facility, you should get good benefits.

Pay ranges I've seen in New York in 2012-2013 from around $16.00 to $25.00/hr. and up. If you work out of a staffing company, the rate may be much higher. (One offered me a $35.00 an-hour contract if I had hospital experience.) Not all northern states pay this well, trust me. Do your research. Some southern states pay very well, like Texas and Georgia. I spoke with several people who worked there and the rate of pay was $15.00 to $20.00 (rates varies, things change), and if you are a traveling technician, $35.00 and up, I heard. All fifty states in the USA have dialysis clinics all over. You can Google pay rates in your state and estimate what to expect. A manager's pay is based on experience, education, and certifications. If you don't have a degree, you can still get/do the job, but a person with a degree is preferred though many times not required. It all depends on what the manager is looking for.

One Common Cash Cow Method

One way is to put in for vacation at your unit for two weeks and go to another private or corporate unit and work normal days over there. You'd just get two separate checks but no overtime because you're employed at two separate unit corporations. The results of this way are good, and a lot of people prefer it because less tax comes out of their check.

Various Feedback Received About My Work Ethics

From Patients

"Gee, girl, you're fast and professional!"

"When can you come back, because I've never seen this kind of treatment before?"

"Can you teach my technician how to stick and clean my arm appropriately?"

"This girl knows her stuff. She put me on right on time and took me off in a quick way!"

"I need to transfer to whatever unit you are at!"

"Wait a minute, she's here. Whew! Thank God!"

"All technicians should get a lesson from you. These technicians don't clean my arm and I bleed a lot after treatment."

"Thank goodness you're our technician. Whew!"

From Previous Staff/Management

- "You are extremely organized. Can you work more days?"

- "Forget the rest, she's the best. Can she come back?"

- "Thank you for coming. Can you even open our unit sometimes?"

- "Wow. What unit are you from again?"

4 Per-Diem Improvements I Made

1. I started asking about rules concerning clocking out during lunchtime.

2. I began showing my appreciation more by making sure I did a good job when asked to render services at a unit.

3. I became more helpful to other teammates, example: ask a teammate if they need a patient in the treatment chair that's been waiting outside and call them in.

CHAPTER #15
THE STATE IS HERE!

The wrong shortcuts can cost you once stuff hits the fan,
so do the right thing at all times and you'll be relieved.

(This chapter is only my perception of inspections, so check your own state requirements.)

"Oh my goodness, the state is here!" This is the exclamation many dialysis staff say, especially me, when I hear that we're up for inspection that day. I get kind of nervous, because I want to be sure I'm doing what I'm supposed to do, and won't get my team members, or the whole clinic in trouble.

If the nurse gave you the okay to put a patient with low/ high blood pressure, or any other complication, such as shortness of breath, on the machine, you SHOULD document this, along with the time and name of the nurse. Many times, dialysis staff gives normal saline or other intervention help to a patient but forgets to document it. This is so serious. Again, documentation is very important; it doesn't matter who you're buddy-buddy with, once the state is there, trust me—document! One thing about the state inspectors, if you're doing what you should be doing, they won't cite the clinic for violations, or close the clinic.

The state can show up any time of the day, walk into the unit, and observe how you care for patients, how you conduct tests in the water treatment room, and much more.

Many times, if the clinic isn't doing what it should, and it looks really bad to the state inspectors, they can close that clinic that day and hour and transfer all the patients to another clinic. If a clinic gets cited for a few minor issues, that clinic has a chance to get it right within a certain time frame before the inspectors return. If the clinic fails to get it right, it possibly can be closed and the person in charge of rectifying the issues is fired.

Some basic reasons why the state comes:

- That clinic is due for a visit, or a revisit to see that the citations have been rectified. All health facilities are subject to government-mandated inspections at regular intervals.

- The clinic has a high death rate or other issues about which they've been notified.

- Patient complaints.

- A new clinic has opened and is due for inspection.

- Other situations.

Some things for which the state can cite you or question you:

- Blood on chair, floor, machines, or anywhere in your area. Even a spot is a big no-no. A lot of trouble can come if you don't clean your patient's area properly. Also, any dried blood on your chair, machine, or area is a trouble sign.

- Improper cleaning of area/machine and chairs.

- Counter cluttered with unnecessary supplies.

- Not familiar with or instructed in doing the chlorine/chloramines test.

- Not being familiar with B/P limits. (For example, you could be asked, "Would you put a patient on with the following blood pressure: 190/110, pulse 90; or 70/50, pulse 80? How high is high and how low is low? Whom would you notify about this?")

- Pulling patients who have finished treatment, but are really bleeding from the access sites, out of the treatment stations and pushing another patient into that station.

- Not properly monitoring patients.

- Not properly documenting issues before, during, and after treatment. (For example, you could be asked, "How is the patient feeling before and after treatment? When will you notify the nurse?")

- Handling emergencies. (For example, you could be asked, "What is the Trendelenburg position?")

EXTREME IMPORTANCE!!

Handling the Isolation Area

It's very serious to walk out of the isolation room in your PPE. If the state is still there, forget it!!

Brief reflections

As a newbie, you should:

- Greet those you see while entering the clinic.

- Be as professional as possible in all circumstances.

- Avoid shortcuts—go by policy.

- Put your patients on the machine professionally.

- Know what the state inspectors are looking for in your unit.

- If you need help or don't understand something, always ask.

- Humble yourself if the inspector finds something you're doing wrong. Apologize and ask how you can improve.

- Do everything you can to cover yourself, because once an incident occurs, it all goes back to the documentation.

CHAPTER #16
SIMPLE RIGHTS IN THE UNIT

Knowing your rights gives you authority over any bad situation.

Patients' Rights

Patients have a lot of rights. Many notice, and many others don't understand what rights they have. Honestly, there's nothing like a patient who knows what's up; but some patients flat out abuse their rights by avenging their feelings toward good staff workers and the company. If a patient is really mistreated by a team member, the patient should exercise his or her right to go up the chain of command and report the problem. Some patients are bold and report harsh situations, and some worry about repercussions if they complain about unsatisfactory treatment. It's your job to inform your patients of their rights concerning making a complaint. If you don't know their rights, intercom the clinical manager, or social worker, and inquire. If a patient wants you to intercom or call the clinical manager for an immediate complaint about someone, tell the nurse, if possible, and the nurse, many times, will intervene. If not, do it yourself. If something goes down with that patient and you refused to notify management, your job will surely be on the line that day.

Patients Have the Right:

-To make a written or verbal complaint.

-To refuse treatment medications.

-To refuse certain individuals handling them.

-To reschedule due to circumstances, without being pressured to "come only on their days."

-To refuse resuscitations (please look at their treatment order or consult the nurse). Some patients don't want to be revived if they pass out on the machine, and it can mean a lawsuit if you attempt to do so against their wishes, so beware.

Your Rights

You, as a patient care provider, also have rights, and if things become threatening, please use them. I've had a few cases where patients have cursed and threatened me for no apparent reason and were very noncompliant and rebellious. At the time, management didn't intervene, I didn't know my rights, and nothing was done, period. I should have taken appropriate action, such as calling the police for the violent threats that mentioned shooting my family and me. I now know my rights and take all violent threats seriously. I've outlined below a few rights for both staff and patients. As always, rights vary from company to company, so know them and ask how to handle a patient if the patient wants to complain.

Staff Rights

-To make a written or verbal complaint.

-To call police for violent or dangerous written or verbal threats.

-To request to be moved to a different section to avoid patient confrontation (but never refuse to provide care if the patient starts bleeding and you're nearby—it's against the law.)

-To request another technician to cannulate a patient who is unruly but not threatening.

-To request management to have a meeting with the patient who's causing issues.

Please Note

Again, document in that patient's chart what happened and what was said. If the company wants to review what's going on, you have proof by documentation. If I'm dealing with a case where my request to move to another section due to a disrespectful patient is ignored, I usually keep paper in my locker, and create a paper trail of dates and notations so that I have proof of the time a situation occurred.

CHAPTER #17
PATIENT CONCERNS

Everyone loves a technician who lends a listening ear and combines it with positive action.

Working in different units, I've met patients from all over world who come to those units. Often, they tell me their likes and dislikes and what they want out of dialysis as a whole. I respect them because I always try to put myself in their shoes at all times. I've heard patients say it would be nice if more doctors were in their unit. Some appreciate staff for working hard to help save their lives. A few patients feel that staff treats them like children, or acts bossy with them. Others are tired of complaining and not seeing desired results. I really love all my patients and try my best to make their dialysis treatment as comfortable as possible.

Many patients go through a lot on hemodialysis. They shouldn't have to deal with staff-to-staff issues, attitudes from staff, or environmental problems, like the central air conditioning not working. I always put myself in the patient's position because, when I've been sick, I've been a patient in various hospitals. When I walk into a hospital, I expect to be treated a certain way. If I'm not, many times I'll make a complaint and tell the culprits my complaint in a calm way. I really hate when I have to wait a long time to see the doctor. That's why time is very important to me—I know how it feels.

Some companies are really strict in terms of their protocols because they want to make sure their patients are treated in a topnotch way. Many times, they only listen to the patient. This is very good and very bad at the same time because a few patients will take advantage of it. I've seen instances when the staff was innocent of the deed the patient accused them of but the company, in fear of a lawsuit, accepted the patient's witness even though it was a lie. I do follow up with those patients about complaints regarding my services. I ask them if I've improved, or what I can do to make my service better—and they tell me. That's how you improve: pay attention to complaints, suggestions, and criticism.

25 Things You Should Know

The more knowledge you receive, the farther along you are.

1. Be sure you have a genuine interest in being a hemodialysis technician. True colors show after a while.

2. Without your technician skills, the nurse's duties would be much harder.

3. You are somebody; never let anyone look down on you.

4. If you have issues with management, go in twos or threes to discuss the issues. Bottom line: Always have a witness.

5. If a patient wants to reject the protocol you're using, document and notify the RN or your clinical manager. Because if you do whatever they ask you to do and it's wrong, and you go on vacation and another technician works your section and does things right, big problems will

arise. The patient will say, "Well, X has been doing this for years. Why should you change now?"

6. If you don't get along with another teammate, even though you've tried everything, request to be moved to another section or shift. Don't get arrogant and say "X will learn today who I really am." Keep the peace. Trust me. The drama isn't worth it.

7. A dialysis clinic is not the place to work on impressing any individual or to join any group politics. Seriously, those folks you're talking to about someone else are the same folks talking to others about you. Don't be fooled!

8. Never—I repeat, never—bring any patient into your feud with any technician or nurse, because if you mess up their arm, they can and will turn on you and tell the tech or nurse all you said that was bad about them.

9. Don't be a person who's selfish and not a team player. You'll need help, and I still appreciate it when I get it. Turnover can be a crazy time some days.

10. If you're an emotional type who breaks down when you hear of the death of a patient, tell your teammates not to mention this to you early in the morning. Ask them to wait until you're on break or going home. It does affect one's day.

11. With each year that passes, protocols and procedures change. Keep yourself up-to-date.

12. Check with some access centers (centers that create access lifelines) to see if they have a program where you can learn about how they fix accesses.

13. Your boss can be your best confidant or your worst enemy.

14. Don't bite the hands of the different centers that feed you with per diem assignments, because you may need extra days in the future.

15. You can never get rid of a hater, but you can do better and accomplish more than one dream if you put your goals together.

16. Patients first, computers next—or last.

17. Never discriminate against any person regardless of their gender, religion, sex, or nationality. It can earn you a pink slip in the mail.

18. Be a positive technician and learn things that will make you the best; read books on thinking and succeeding.

19. Don't make people regret their decision to hire you, or invite you to their unit to do per diem .

20. If you open the unit, be sure you check your logbook correctly and know the chlorine/chloramines test by heart because the state often asks the openers how they do their job the correct way.

21. Tempted to do wrong? Be reminded that you can and will get caught. Replacing a technician is easy, and so is replacing a nurse. The difference is, the nurse has a nursing degree and can get another job rather quickly, while you, on the other hand, will be banned from the dialysis clinics with no nursing degree in hand.

22. Educate yourself at free company classes. That's how I became knowledgeable in this field. I went to every dialysis class I could.

23. If you see a patient being abused by a staff member—like sexual harassment, or verbal abuse to the elderly—do not be silent.

24. Be humble, but don't be a dummy for anyone. You mean something, but don't do too much outside your job description.

25. Be a real team player. Don't be a selfish, all-about-me technician. Find a teammate who's the same and work together.

REFLECTIONS

Thank you for reading this book.

Looking back over every chapter makes many of my past experiences feel as if they happened yesterday; indeed, seven years went by very fast. As you have read, I've gone through a lot—even a bit more than I conveyed here. If I could get a job in dialysis when I knew nothing about dialysis, you surely can. I'll always suggest thinking positive and going for it. I feel it's very important early on to decide if you want to make the dialysis field a career because you really don't want to spend your whole workday in a place you can't stand. Honestly, I love working in dialysis for the sake and happiness of taking care of my patients, but it can get crazy.

What made me write this book is the hard times. This uncommon idea dropped in my heart in the year 2012. I remembered how much I had gone through and how I turned it around. I had some really rough moments, days, and weeks, which turned into months of turmoil dealing with rumors, hateful people, doing my job totally correctly, coworker and patient issues, and so much more. It took me years to forgive others and bury the hurt caused by the different events that I encountered in the dialysis world. I managed to get through it and because of those situations I am a much better person. I truly wish I'd had a book like this before I started in the dialysis field. Through it all, I managed to work through those issues and share with others what working in dialysis is all about.

To those who are in the field and love it, keep your head up. If you've read this book and haven't gotten the job, continue to press on. As long as you have faith that you'll get it, you will. If you're in a tough dialysis environment and are tired of your situation, it's time to get out that notepad and pen, write down your dreams, and make them happen. So, in conclusion, I encourage you to set the record straight by making the right decisions now so that you and your future generations can greatly benefit. I hope this book has helped you in some way! Thanks for reading it.

Top Companies That Hire Dialysis Technicians

Fresenius Medical Center

http://jobs.fmcna.com/

Davita

http://careers.davita.com/

Gambro

http://www.gambro.com/

American Renal

http://www.americanrenal.com/

Favorite Health Care

https://www.favoritestaffing.com

DSI Renal

http://www.dsi-corp.com/

A list of all Dialysis Centers in all 50 USA states

http://dialysiscenters.org

http://www.dialysisunits.com/

Educational Materials

Books on Amazon

The Wisdom Secret Diary of a Dialysis Technician

Websites (learning about nephrology and dialysis)

The National Kidney Foundation

http://www.kidney.org/professionals/cnnt/techcnnt.cfm

The American Society of Nephrology (ASN)

http://www.asn-online.org/

Nephrology Clinical Solutions (NCS) (Improves the impact of nephrology therapies and patient care through education, training, and clinical solutions.) http://nephrologyclinicalsolutions.com

Dialysis Training

http://dialysistechnicianstraining.com

Connect With Cassia For More Dialysis Tips

Below are ways you can stay in touch with the latest expert tips from me.

For information, Contact **Cassia Ann**

Through my **blog**
www.dialysistechniciansworldwide.blogspot.com

Connect with Cassia Ann via **YouTube**, **Twitter** and **Facebook**

YouTube:

https://www.youtube.com/Mzconspikulous

Twitter

https://www.twitter.com/dialysistechs

Facebook Fan Page for this book

https://www.facebook.com/DTechsUSA

I created a total of 4 Facebook Groups

Only Dialysis Technician & Staff group

https://www.facebook.com/groups/dialysistechsww

(I handed the group to a new admin but it is still a great group with over 6k members).

POWER GROUP (I handed the group to a new admin, still good group over 2k members).

https://www.facebook.com/groups/1417405875004281/?ref=share

Experienced Dialysis Technicians Only (group only for dialysis technicians with over one year of experience).

https://www.facebook.com/groups/1886177211697278

CCHT/BONENT (This group was created for people looking to study for the CCHT/BONENT. Nurses are welcomed in this group).

https://www.facebook.com/groups/146721199373914/

Dialysis Nurses Rock PERIOD (A group for new and seasoned dialysis nurses/managers).

https://www.facebook.com/groups/WEDNRP

Valuable information

Certified School & Program Directory

More information is available via http://www.bonent.org
The CCHT website is http://www.nncc-exam.org for
information on their certification.

INTERNATIONAL

INDIA
Nephrocare Health Services Pvt. Ltd
1st Floor, West Wing, Punnaiah Plaza,
Above SBI, Road Number 2, Banjara Hills,
Near Jubilee Hills Check Post,
Hyderabad, Telangana 500034, India
Phone: +91 95-50-198899
Fax: +91-40-40184120
Website: www.nephroplus.com

NATIONAL

NMTSC Detachment Portsmouth
Hemodialysis Technician School
1001 Holcomb Road
Portsmouth, VA 23708-5200
Phone: (757) 825-2947

Online Programs

Utopia Health Career Center
(Online Program)
1088 Plaza Drive

Kissimmee, FL 34743
Phone: (407) 962-0299
Website: www.utopiahcc.com

Heritage Health Career Center
(Online Program)
900 S Westover Blvd, Suite A
Albany, GA 31721
Phone: (229) 496-1047
Website: http://heritagehcc.com

Career Step, LLC
(Online Program)
2901 North Ashton Blvd
Suite 101
Lehi, UT 84043
Phone: (800) 411-7073
Website: www.careerstep.com

Arizona

Pima Medical Institute
2160 S. Power Road
Mesa, AZ 85209
Phone: (480) 898-9898
Fax: (480) 641-4522
Website: www.pmi.edu

California

Dialysis Education Services, LLC
16925 Bellflower Blvd
Bellflower, CA 90706
Phone: (562) 376-4181

Fax: (562) 376-4186
Website: www.dialysiseducationservices.org

Florida
Active Health Institute
6520 W Flagler St
Miami, FL 33144-2920
Phone: (305) 648-3293
Fax: (305) 648-3294
Website: www.ahimiami.com

American College of Health and Sciences
2800 N State Road 7
Margate, FL 33063
Phone: (954) 802-8100
Website: www.americancollegefl.org

Emberlynn Hills Academy
(Hemodialysis Patient Care Technician Training)
220 Congress Park Drive, Suite 240
Delray Beach, FL 33445
Phone: (561) 600-0051
Website: www.eha.academy

Emberlynn Hills Academy
(Nurse Training Program)
220 Congress Park Drive, Suite 240
Delray Beach, FL 33445
Phone: (561) 600-0051
Website: www.eha.academy

Floridian Institute
(Hemodialysis Patient Care Technician Training)
13980 SW 47th St
Miami, FL 33175-4404

Phone: (786) 717-6461
Website: www.floridianinstitute.org

Floridian Institute
(Nurse Training Program)
13980 SW 47th St
Miami, FL 33175-4404
Phone: (786) 717-6461
Website: www.floridianinstitute.org

NorthStar University Career Center
2925 E South Street
Orlando, FL 32803
Phone: (407) 780-0759
Website: www.northstaruniversity.net

Utopia Health Career Center
(Hemodialysis Patient Care Technician Training)
1088 Plaza Drive
Kissimmee, FL 34743
Phone: (407) 962-0299
Website: www.utopiahcc.com

Utopia Health Career Center
(Nurse Training Program)
1088 Plaza Drive
Kissimmee, FL 34743
Phone: (407) 962-0299
Website: www.utopiahcc.com

Georgia
Central Georgia Technical College
3300 Macon Tech Drive
H Bldg #249
Macon, GA 31206

Phone: (478) 757-3400
Website: www.centralgatech.edu

Illinois
Delmon Medical College, LLC
7301 N Lincoln Ave, Suite 205
Lincolnwood, IL 60712
Phone: (847) 675-6295

Midwestern Career College
203 North LaSalle St. Ste. 1400
Chicago, IL 60601
Website: www.MCcollege.edu

Tukiendorf Training Institute
5310 N. Harlem Avenue., Suite 209
Chicago, IL 60656
Phone: (773) 774-2222
Fax: (773) 545-7139
Website: www.TTIMedicalSchool.com

Indiana

Duke Training Institute, LLC
120 E Market Street, Suite 808
Indianapolis, IN 46204
Phone: (800) 566-3880
Website: www.duketraininginstitute.com

New Jersey

Branford Institute
302 Main St Fl 2
Paterson, NJ 07505

Phone: 973-881-9428
Website: www.branfordinstitute.org

Camden County College
200 College Dr
Blackwood, NJ 08012-3228
Phone: (856) 374-4902
Fax: (856) 374-4866
Website: www.camdencc.edu

Hudson County Community College
161 Newkirk St, Rm E504
Jersey City, NJ 07306-3006
Phone: (201) 360-4239
Fax: (856) 374-4866
Website: www.hccc.edu/continuing-education/health/

New York

Access Careers - Brooklyn
25 Elm Pl, Ste 201
Brooklyn, NY 11201-5826
Phone: (718) 643-9060
Website: www.accesscareers.edu/

Queensborough Community College
(Continuing Education & Workforce Development)
222-05-56th Avenue
L-118-P
Bayside, NY 11364
Website: www.qcc.cuny.edu/conted

Dialysis Training Institute of Excellence, LLC
831 Merrick Rd

Baldwin, NY 11510-3331
Phone: (516) 705-4637
Website: www.dtietraining.com

HHD Renal Consultant and Service, Inc.
952 Carmans Road
Massapequa, NY 11758
Phone: (917) 913-2218

New York Medical Career Training Center
500 8th Ave Fl 5
New York, NY 10018
Phone: (212) 947-4444
Fax: (646) 596-8022
Website: www.NYmedtraining.com

New York Medical Career Training Center
3609 Main St, Fl 5
Flushing, NY 11354
Phone: (917) 609-3880
Fax: (718) 539-9655
Website: www.nymedtraining.com

Ohio

Centers for Dialysis Care
18720 Chagrin Blvd.
Shaker Heights, OH 44122
Phone: (216) 295-7000 ext. 225
Fax: (216) 295-7014
Website: www.cdcare.org

Excel Career Training Center
12200 Ford Road, Suite 401
Farmers Branch, TX 75234
Phone: (469) 828-1981
Website: excelcareertraining.org

Optimum Dialysis Training Academy
(Hemodialysis Patient Care Technician Training)
101 E Randol Mill Road, #105
Arlington, TX 76011
Phone: (817) 462-0585
Website: optimumdialysistrainingacademy.com

Optimum Dialysis Training Academy
(Nurse Training Program)
101 E Randol Mill Road, #105
Arlington, TX 76011
Phone: (817) 462-0585
Website: optimumdialysistrainingacademy.com

St. Bernadette of Lourdes Training Center
(Hemodialysis Patient Care Technician Training)
12224 Suite B Almeda Road
Houston, TX 77045
Phone: (713) 433-7252
Fax: (713) 433-2222
Website: www.sblchealth.com

St. Bernadette of Lourdes Training Center
(Nurse Training Program)
12224 Suite B Almeda Road
Houston, TX 77045
Phone: (713) 433-7252

Fax: (713) 433-2222
Website: www.sblchealth.com

Utah

Career Step, LLC
2901 North Ashton Blvd
Suite 101
Lehi, UT 84043
Phone: (800) 411-7073
Website: www.careerstep.com

Made in the USA
Monee, IL
16 April 2023

31974074R00098